I0511687

PICTURE BOOK OF

FLOWERS

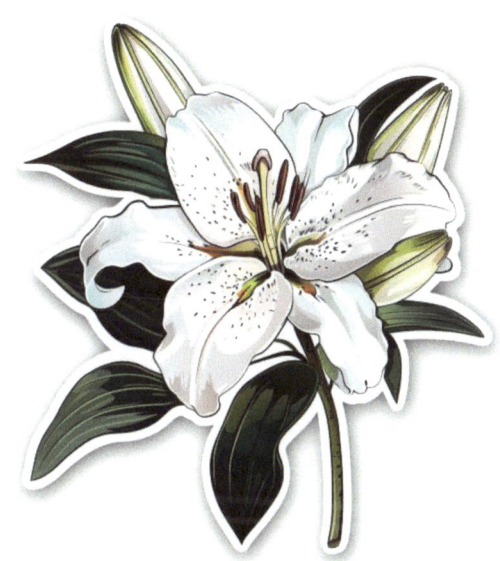

...By...

Ella Caldwell

Copyright © 2024. All rights reserved.

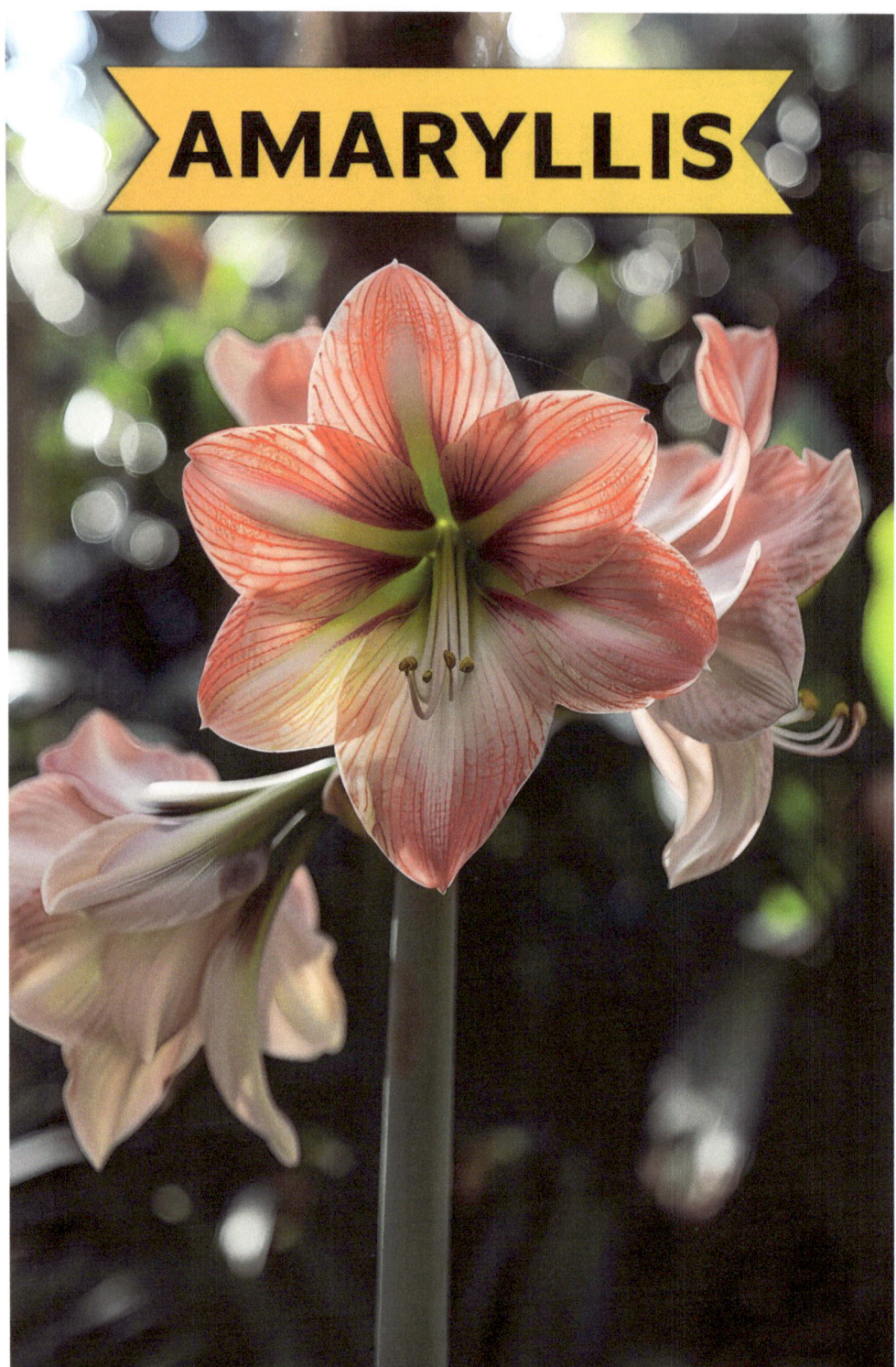

AMARYLLIS

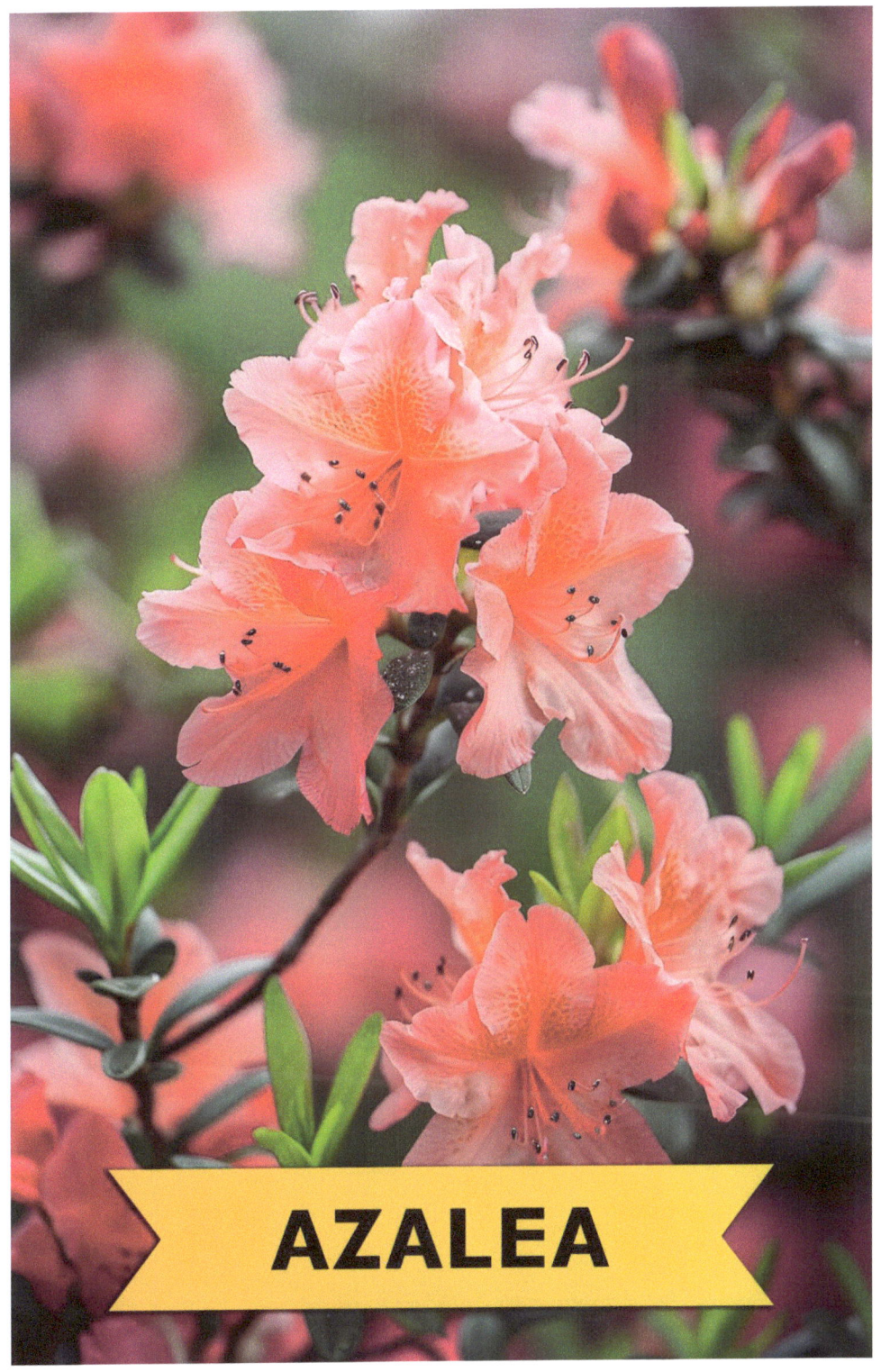

AZALEA

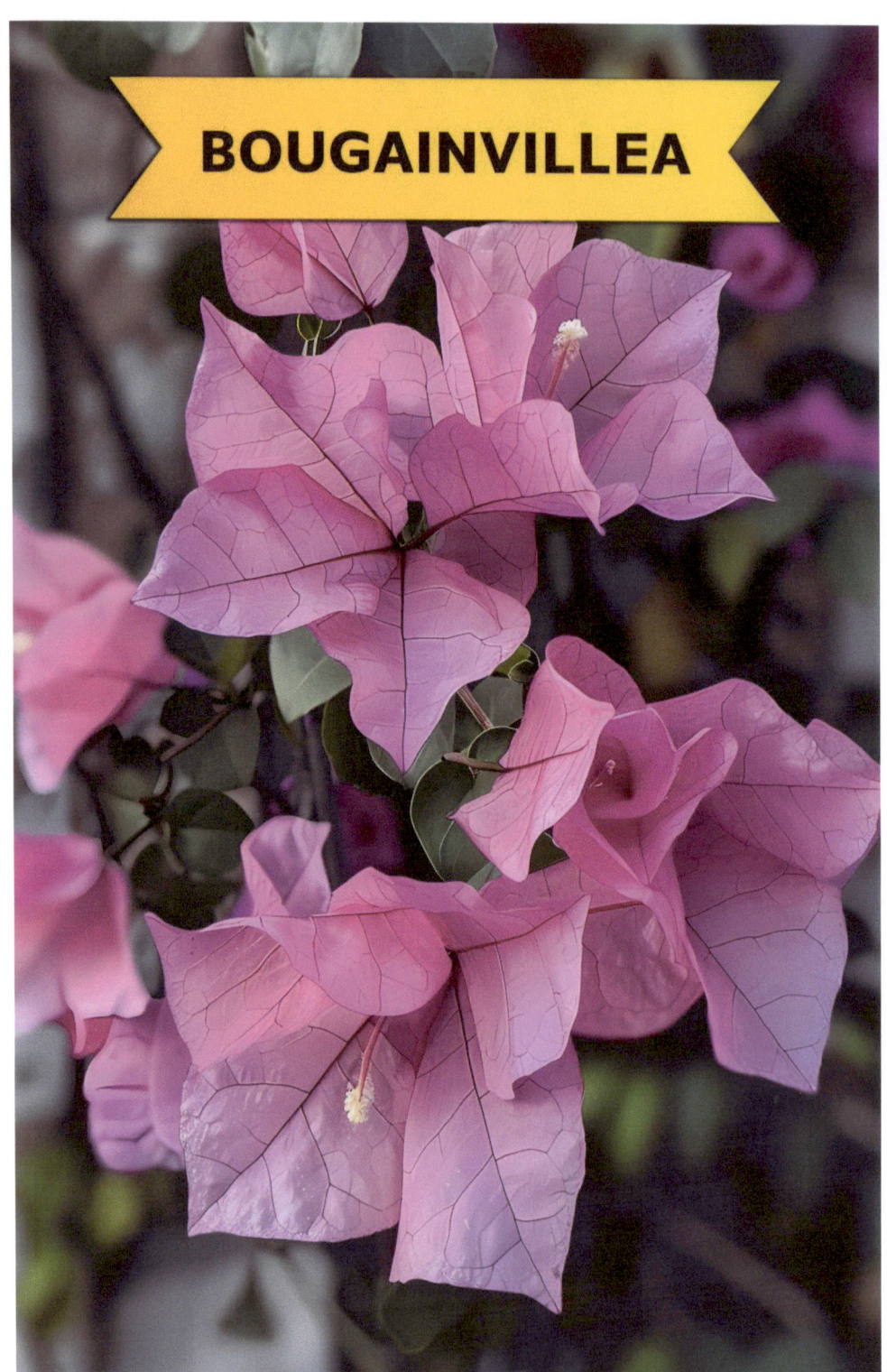

BOUGAINVILLEA

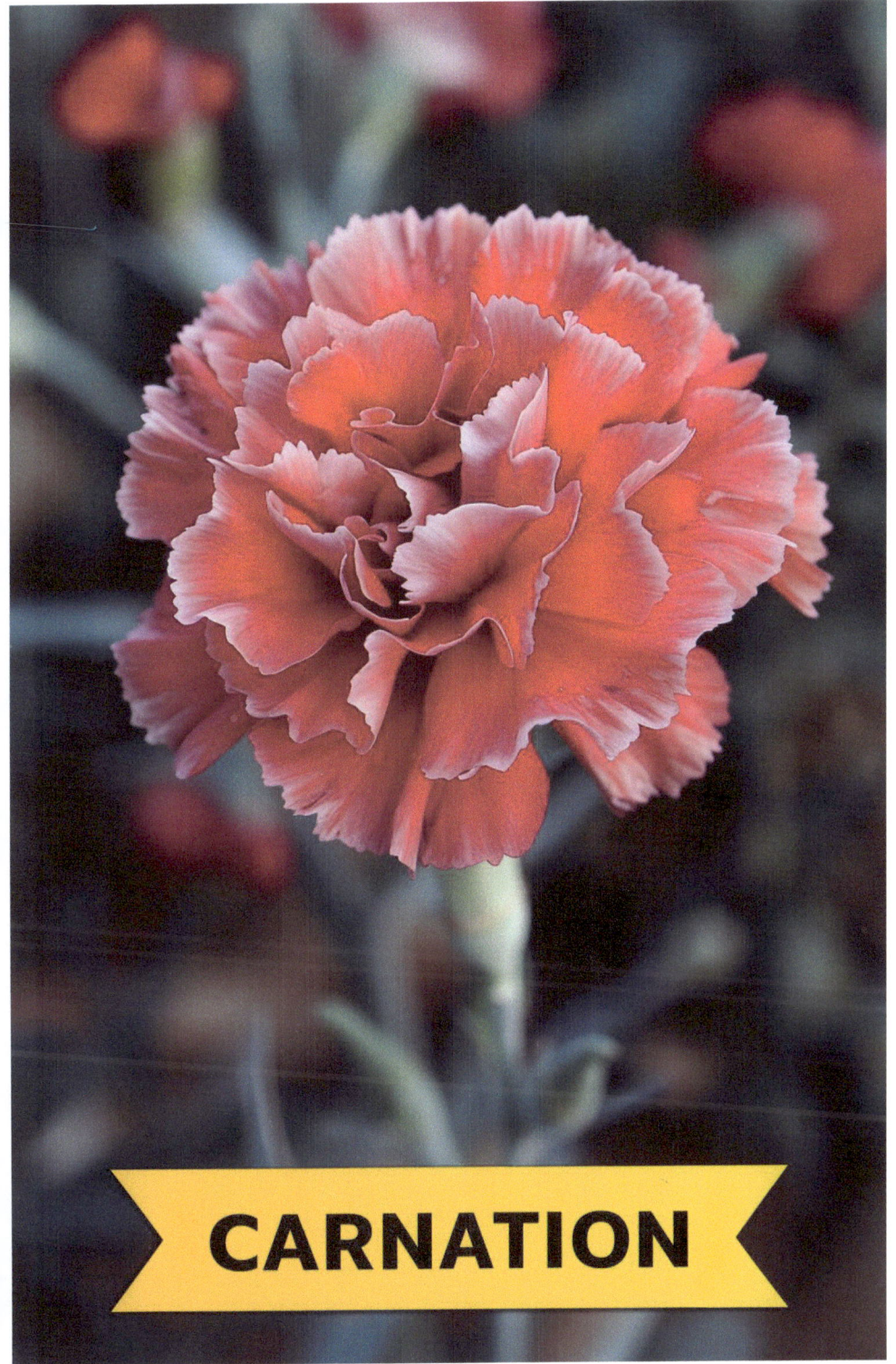

CARNATION

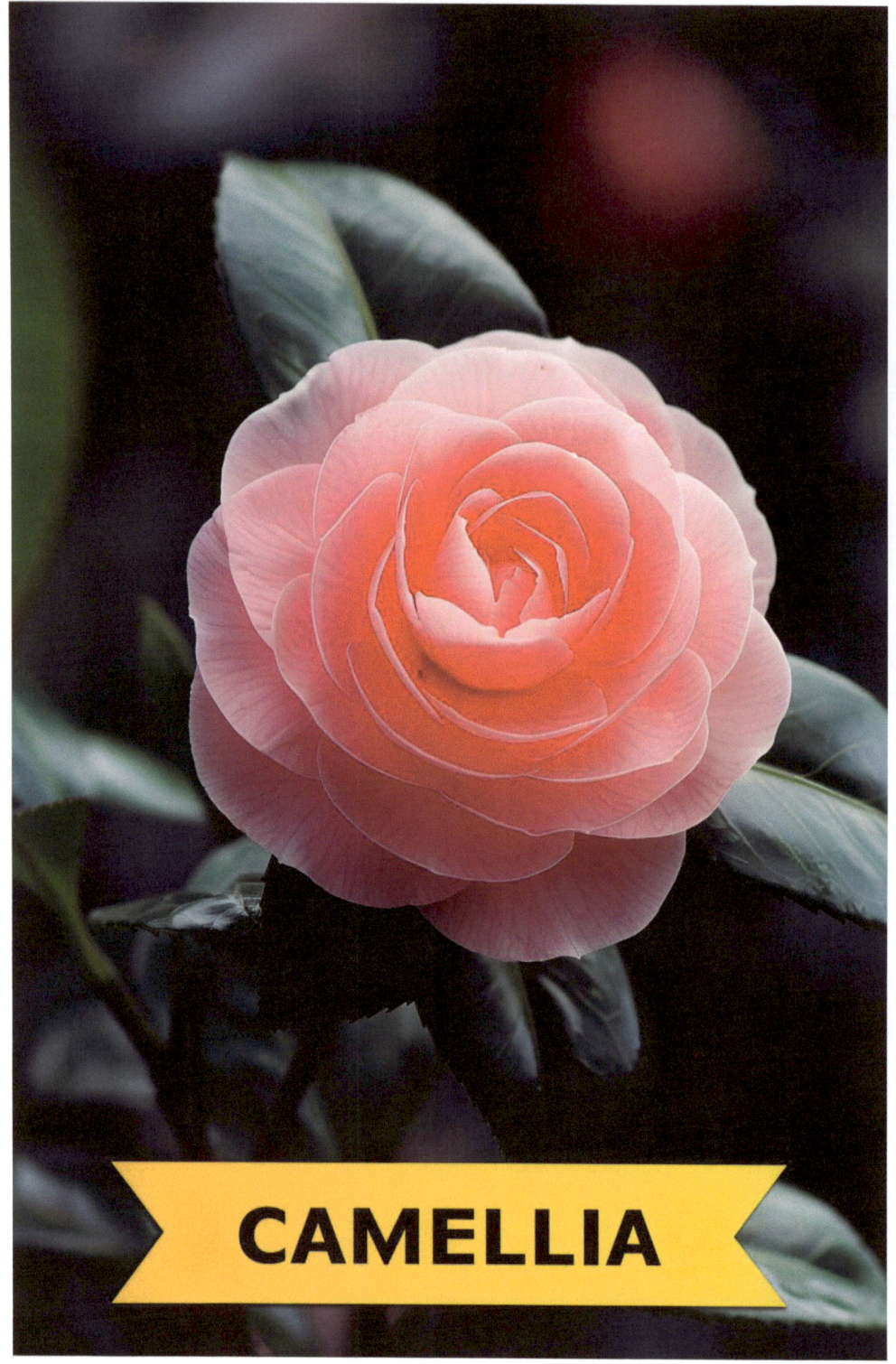

CAMELLIA

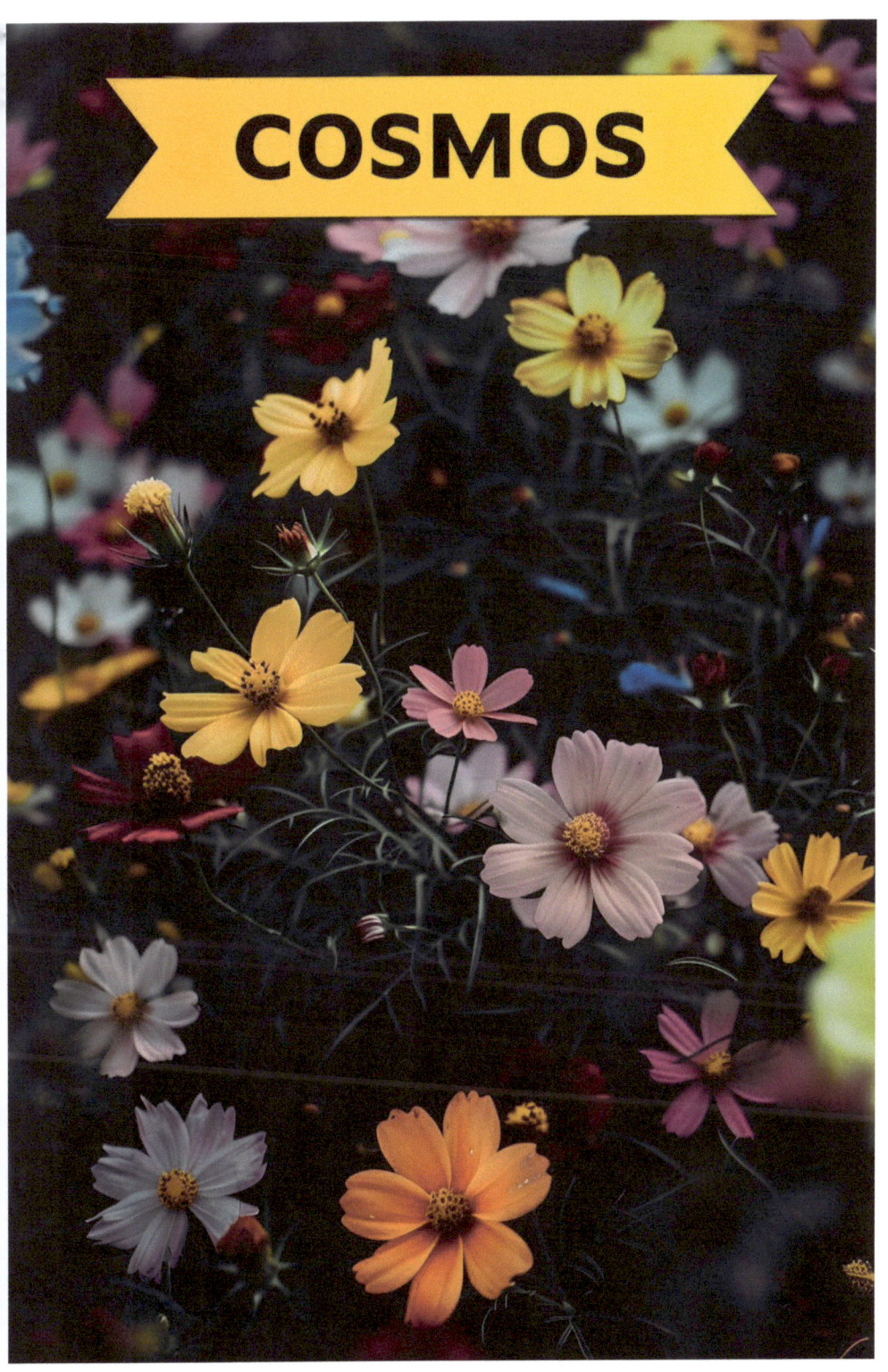

COSMOS

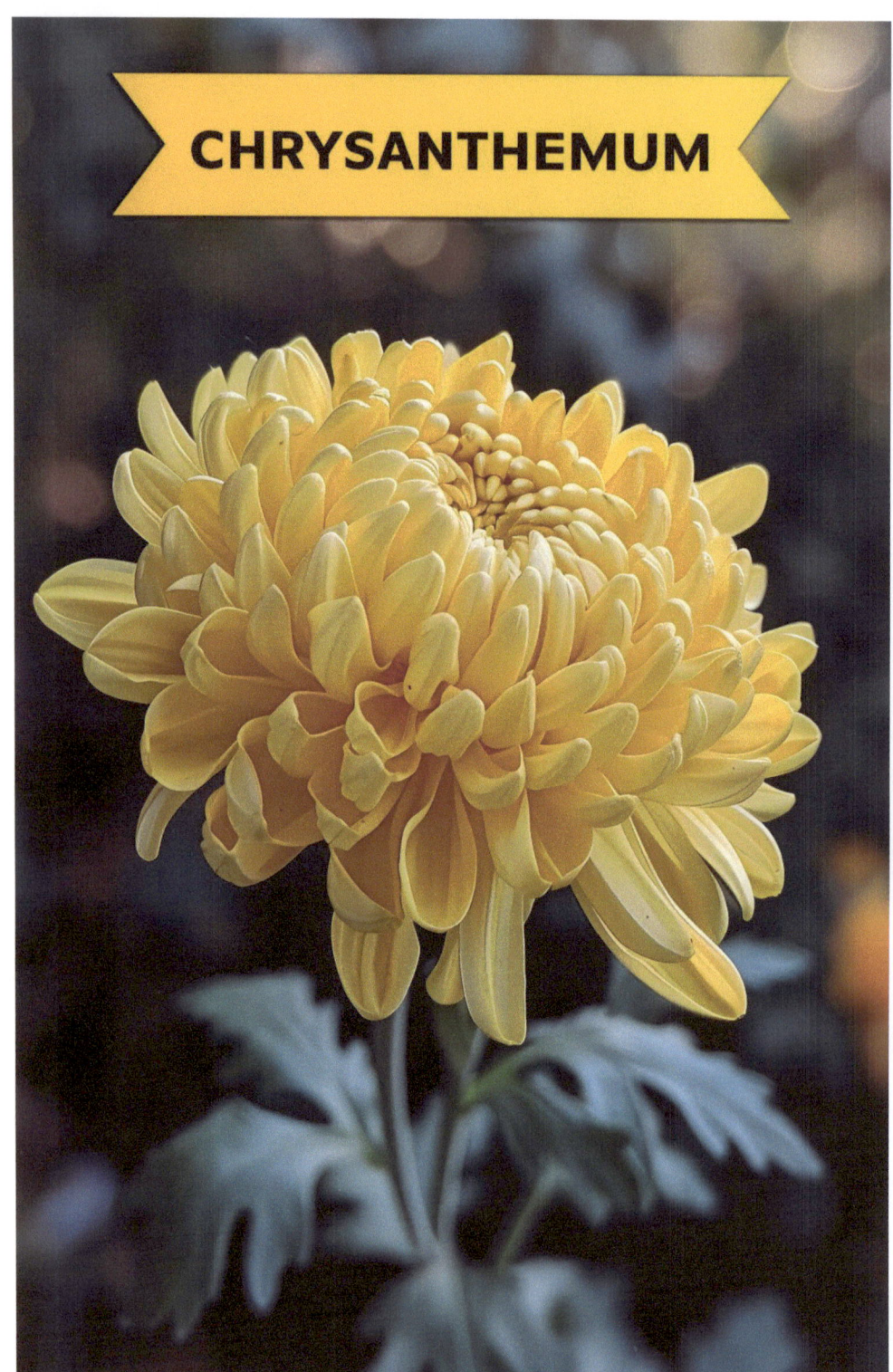

CHRYSANTHEMUM

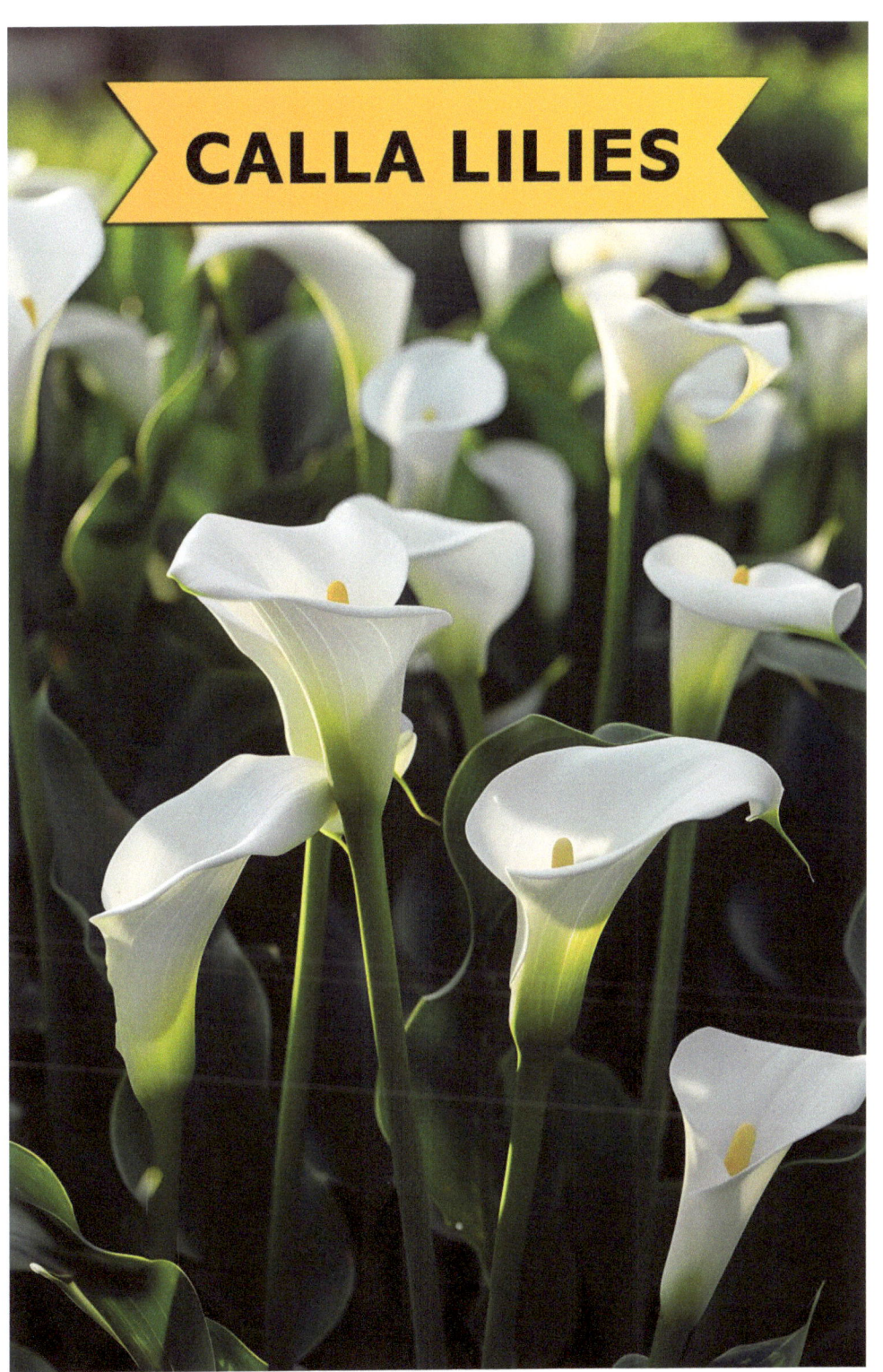

CALLA LILIES

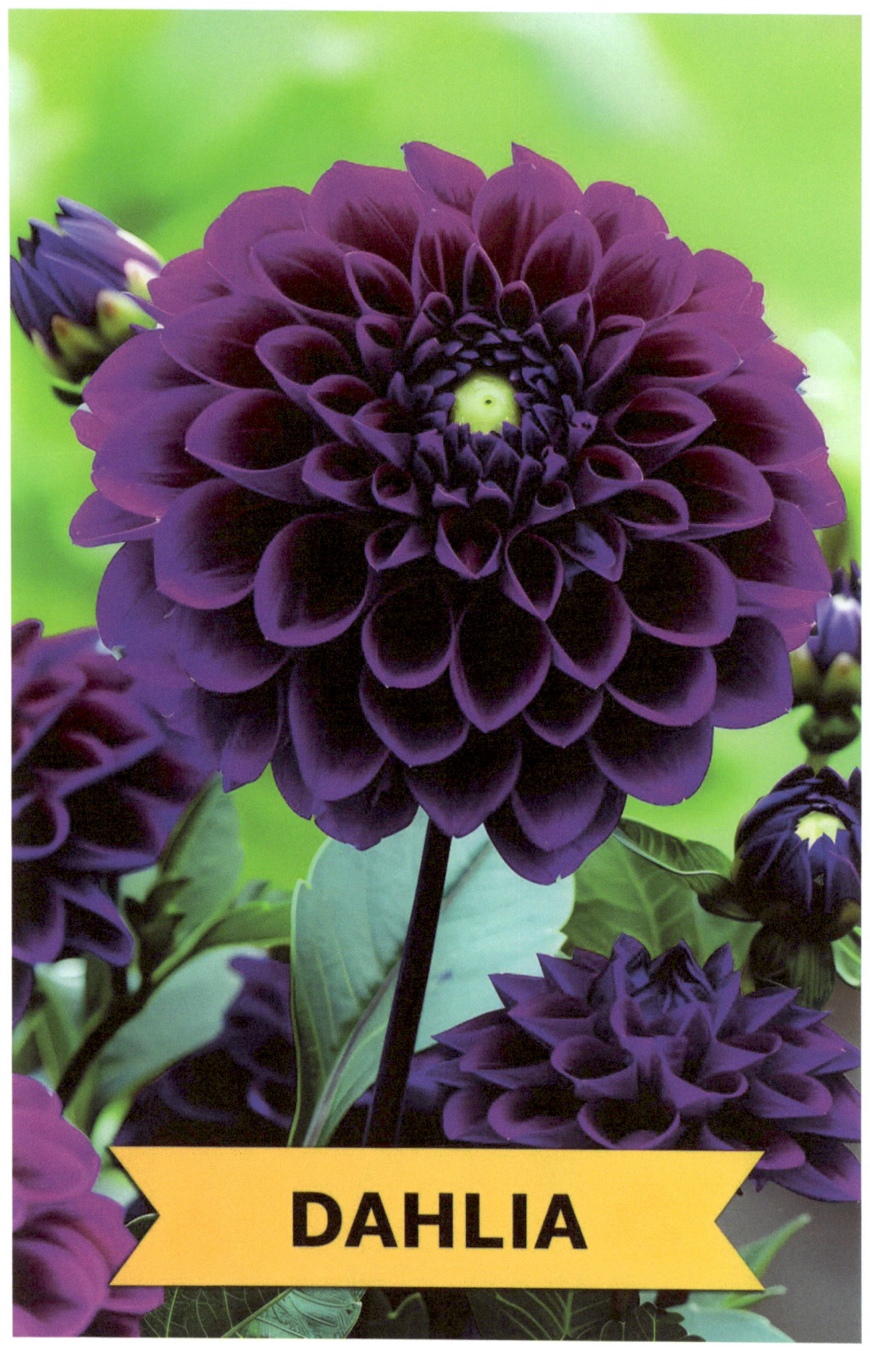

DAHLIA

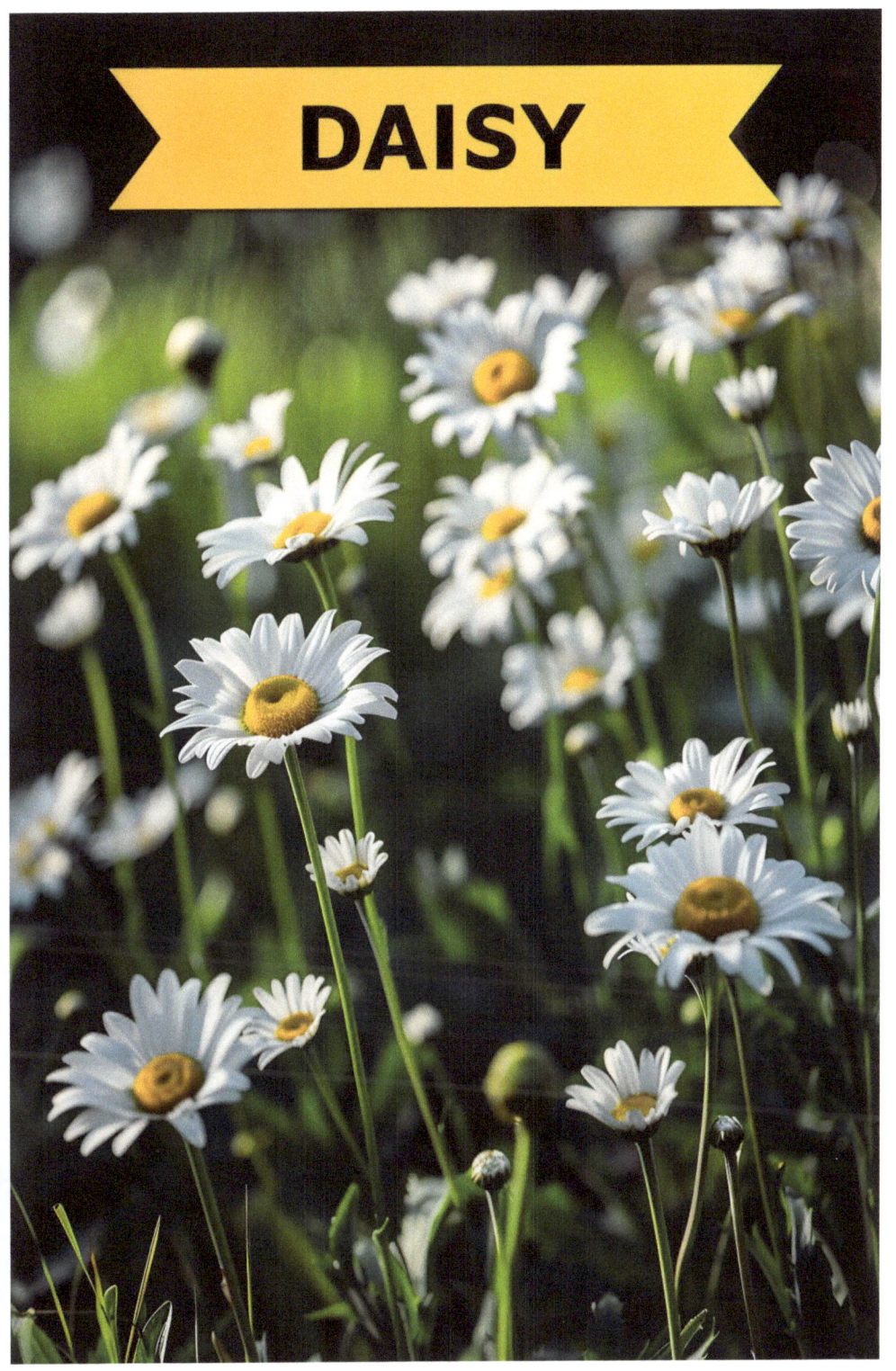

DAISY

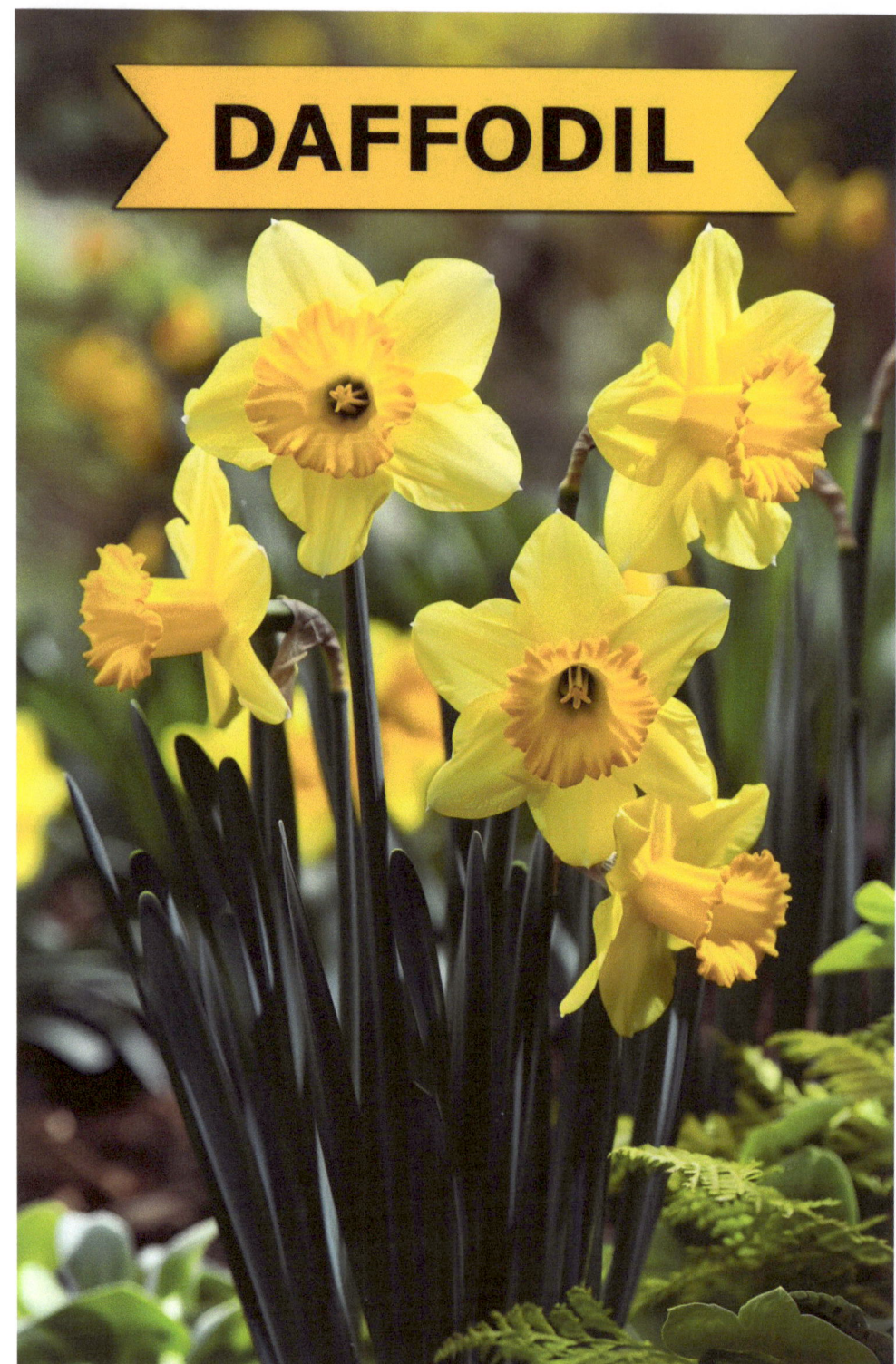

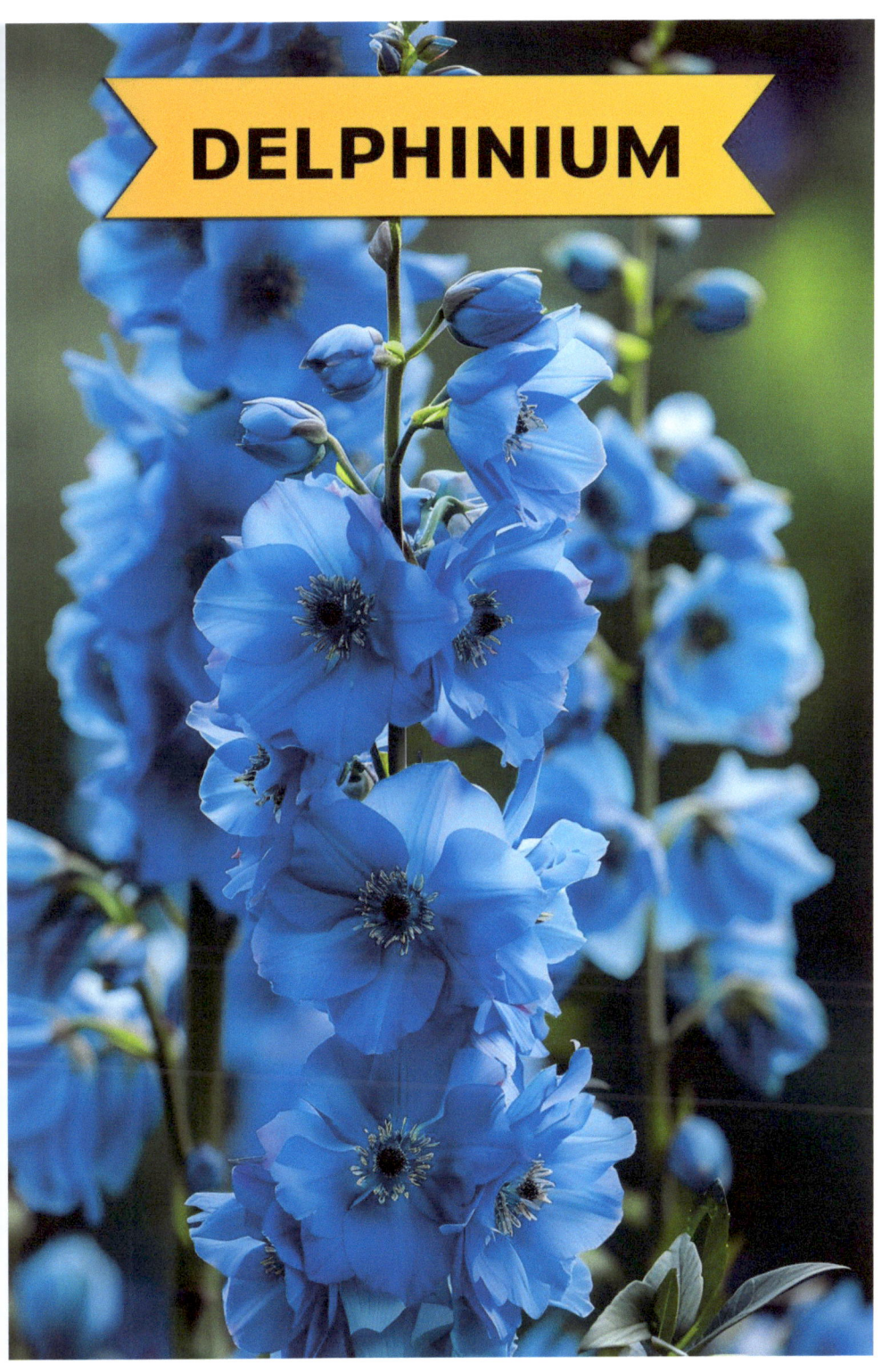

DELPHINIUM

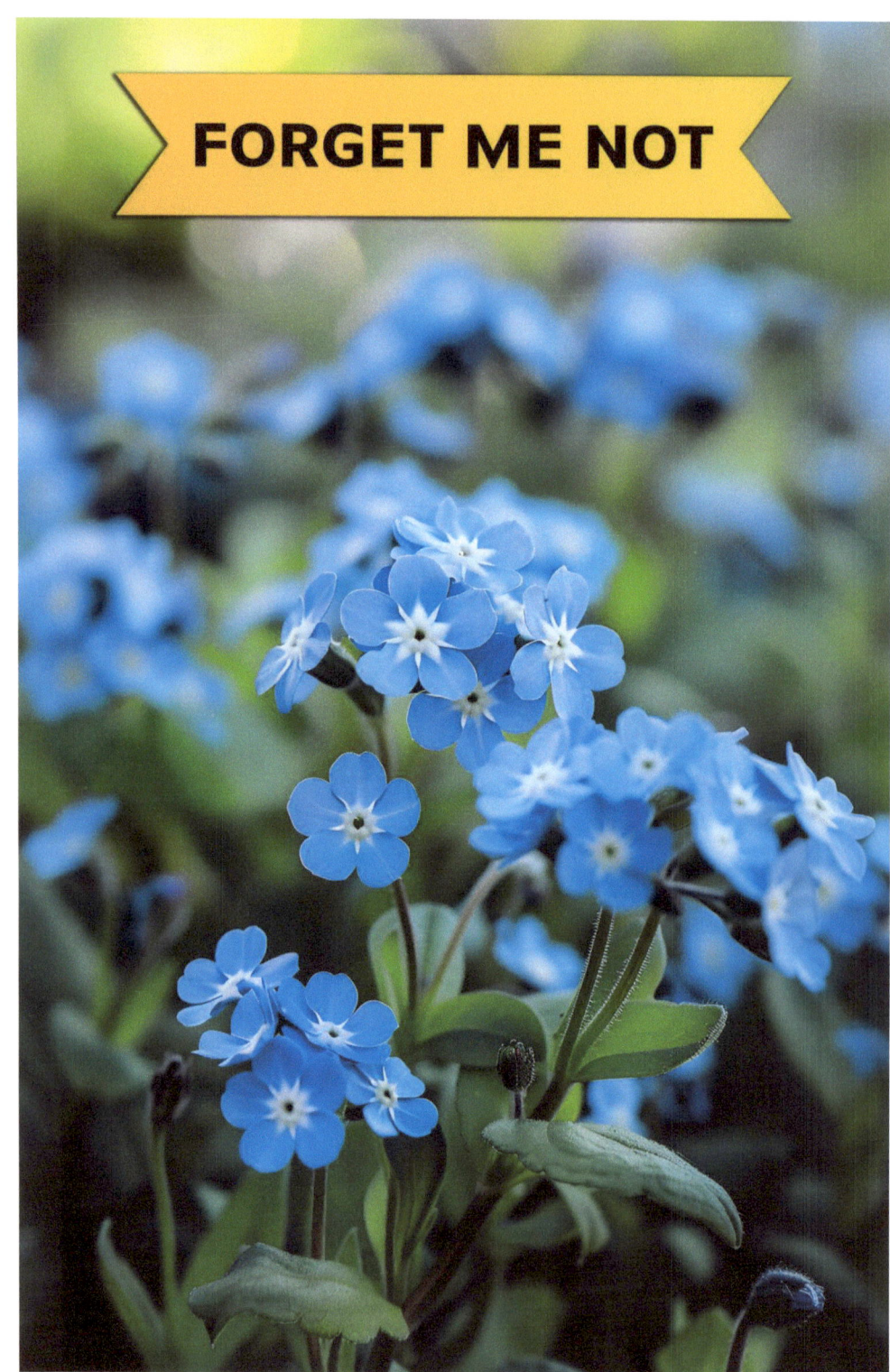

FORGET ME NOT

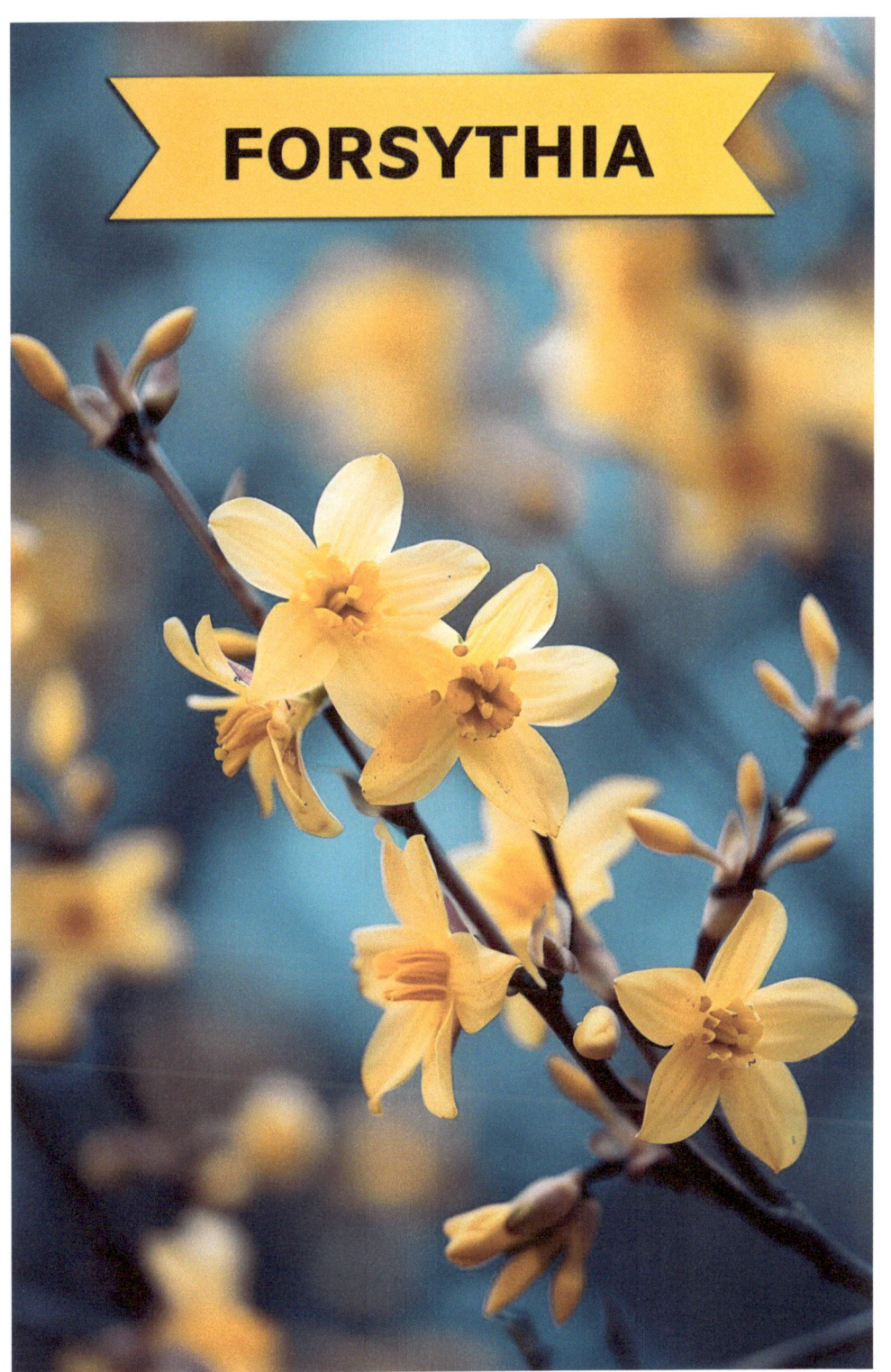

FORSYTHIA

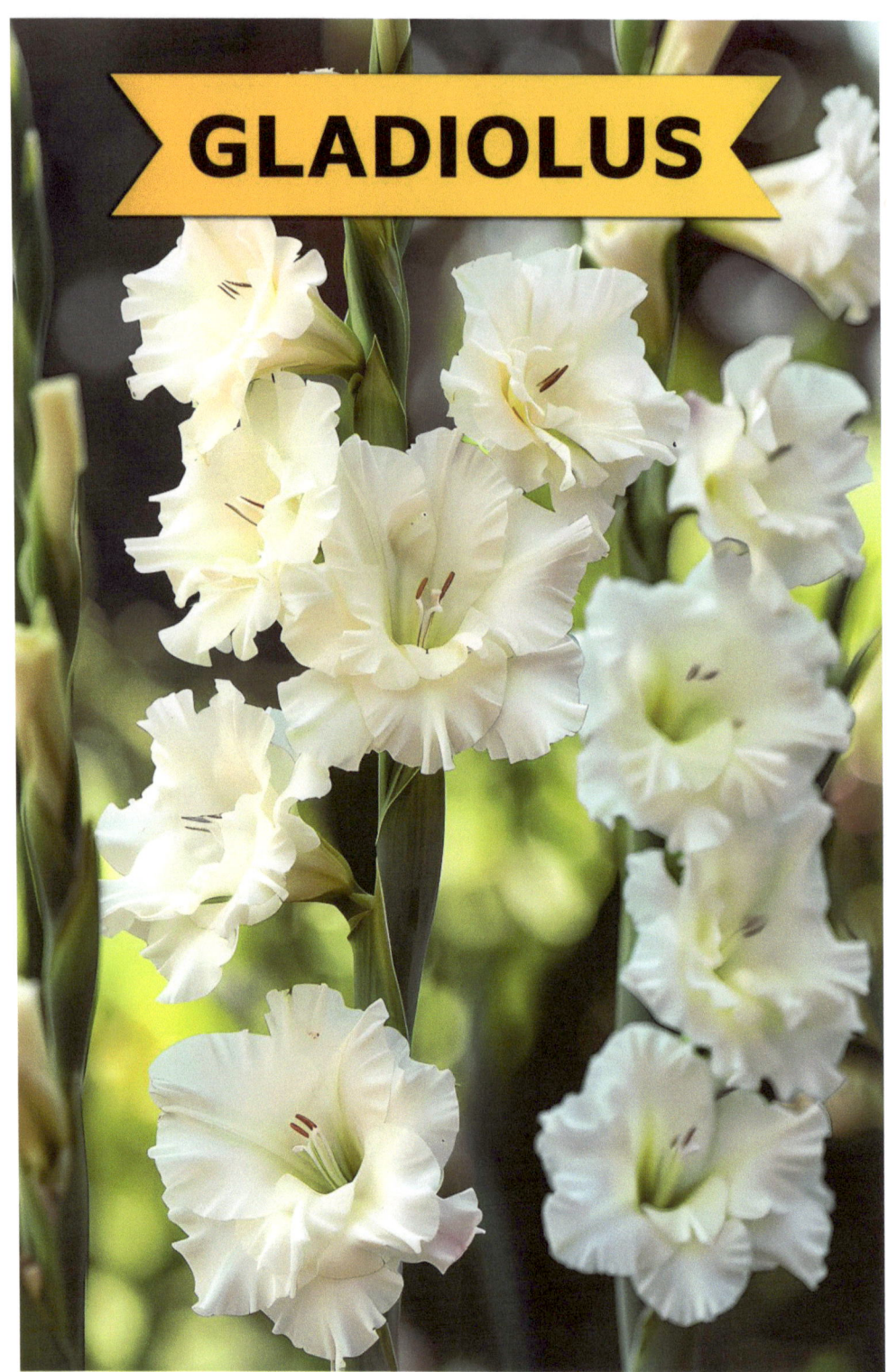

GLADIOLUS

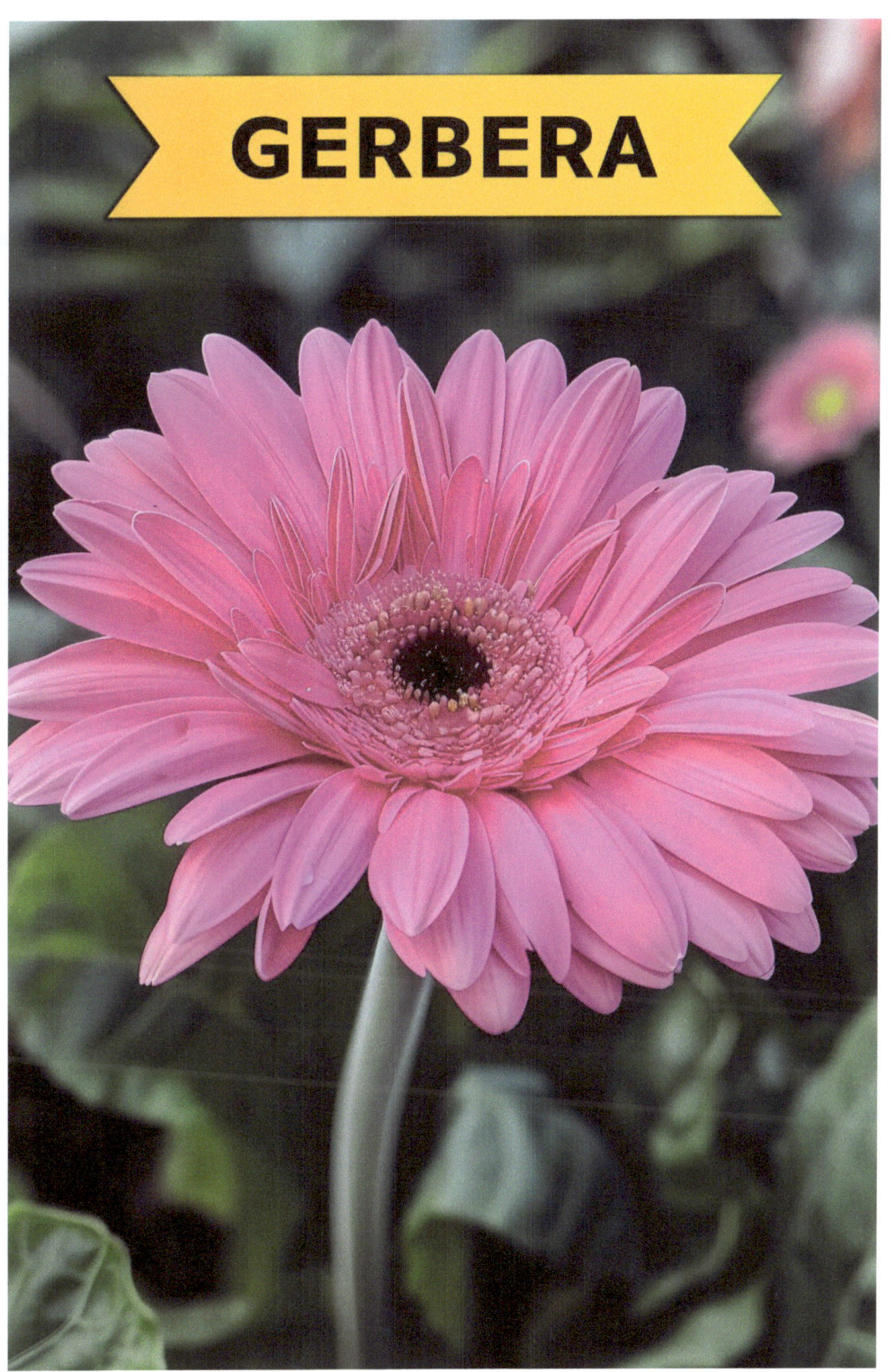

GERBERA

GARDENIA

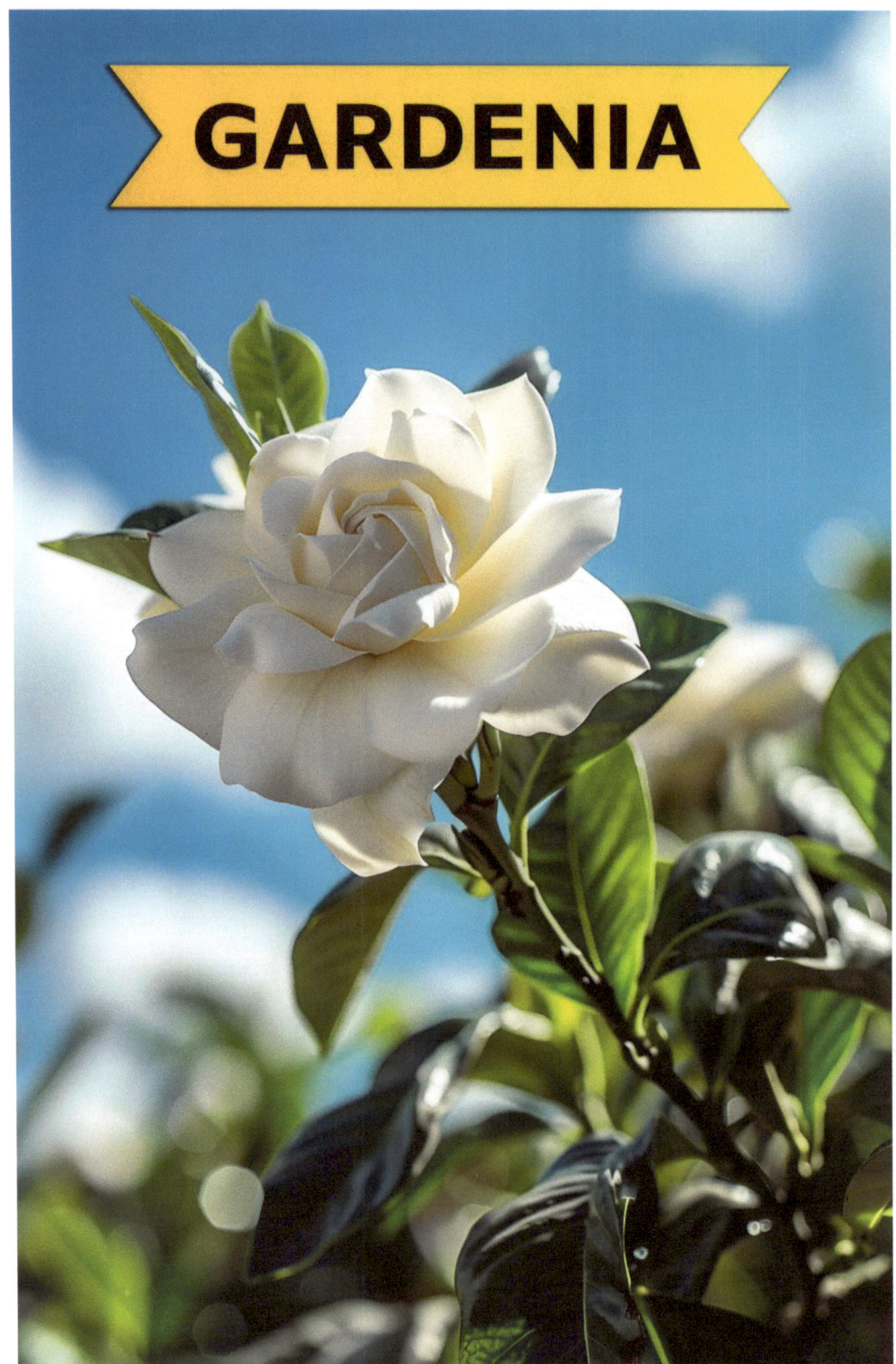

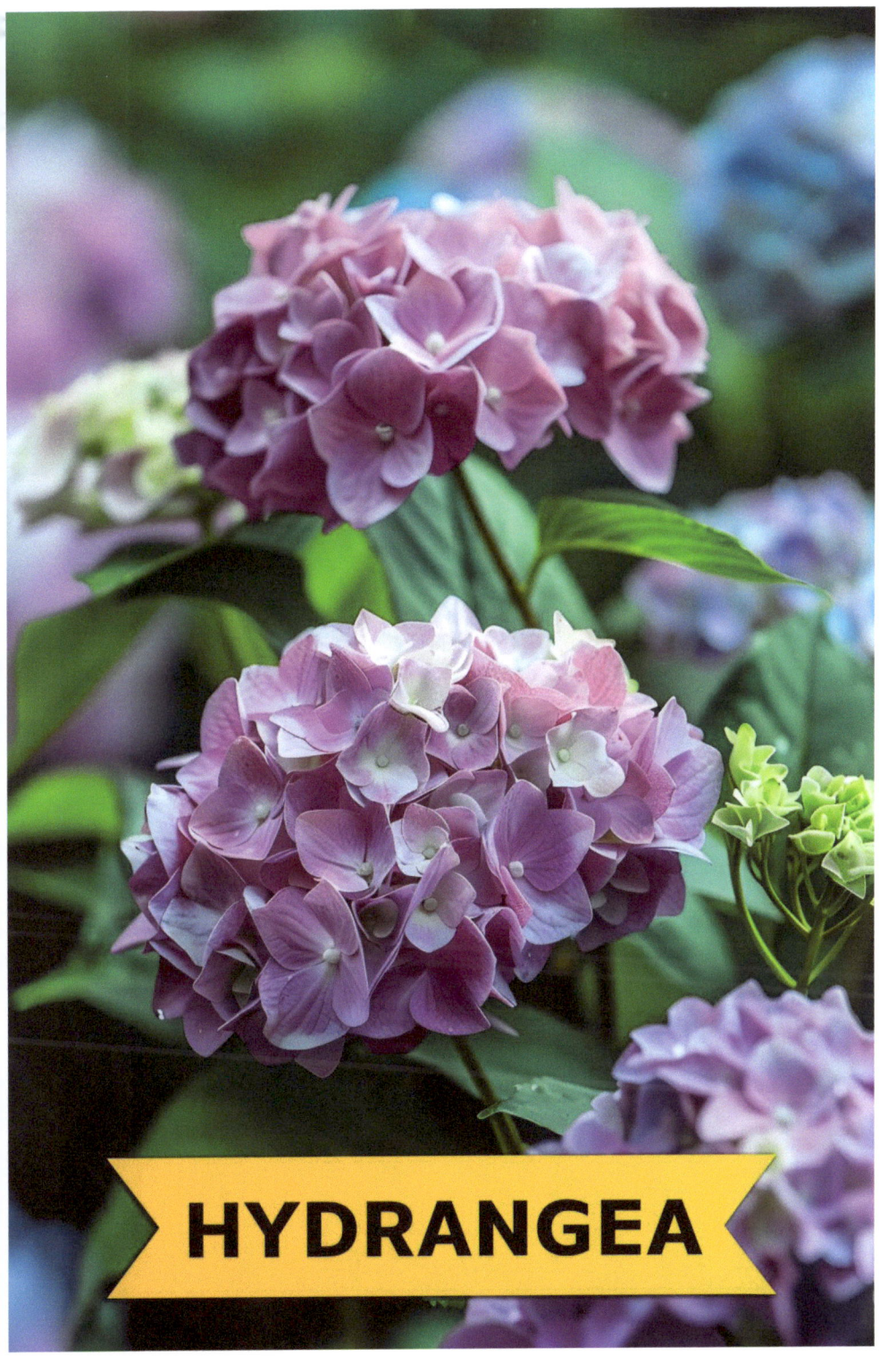

HYDRANGEA

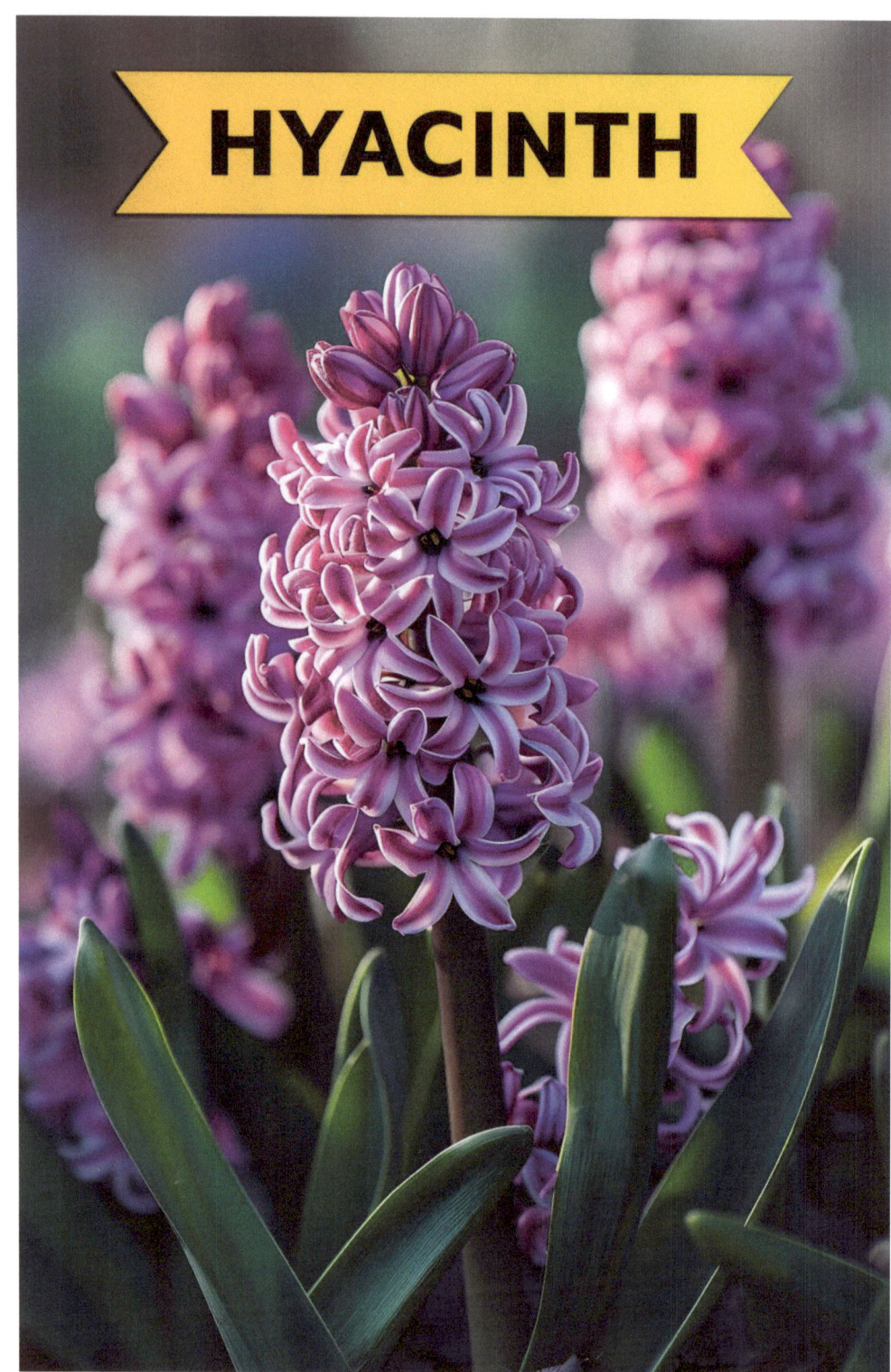

HYACINTH

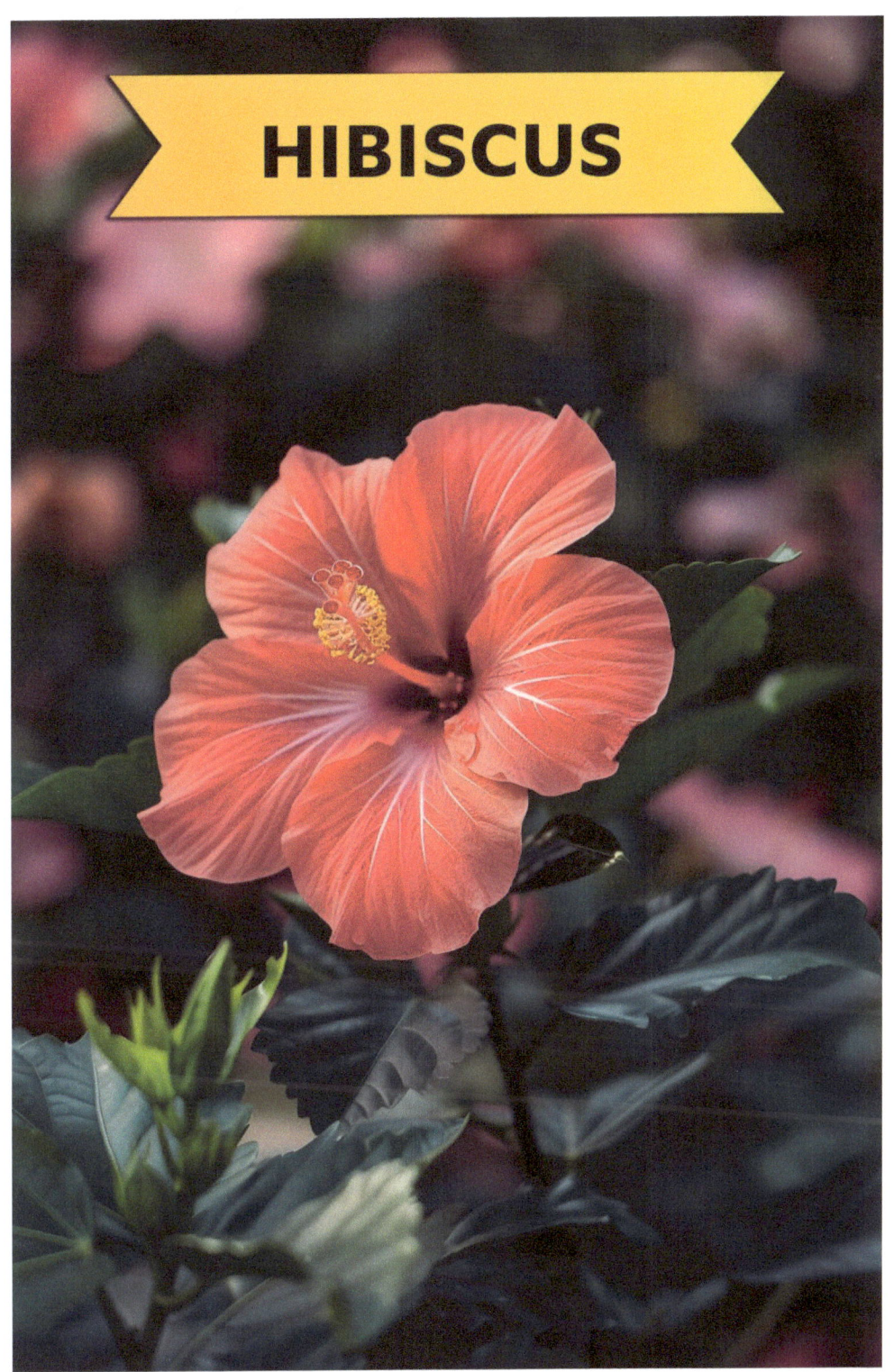

HIBISCUS

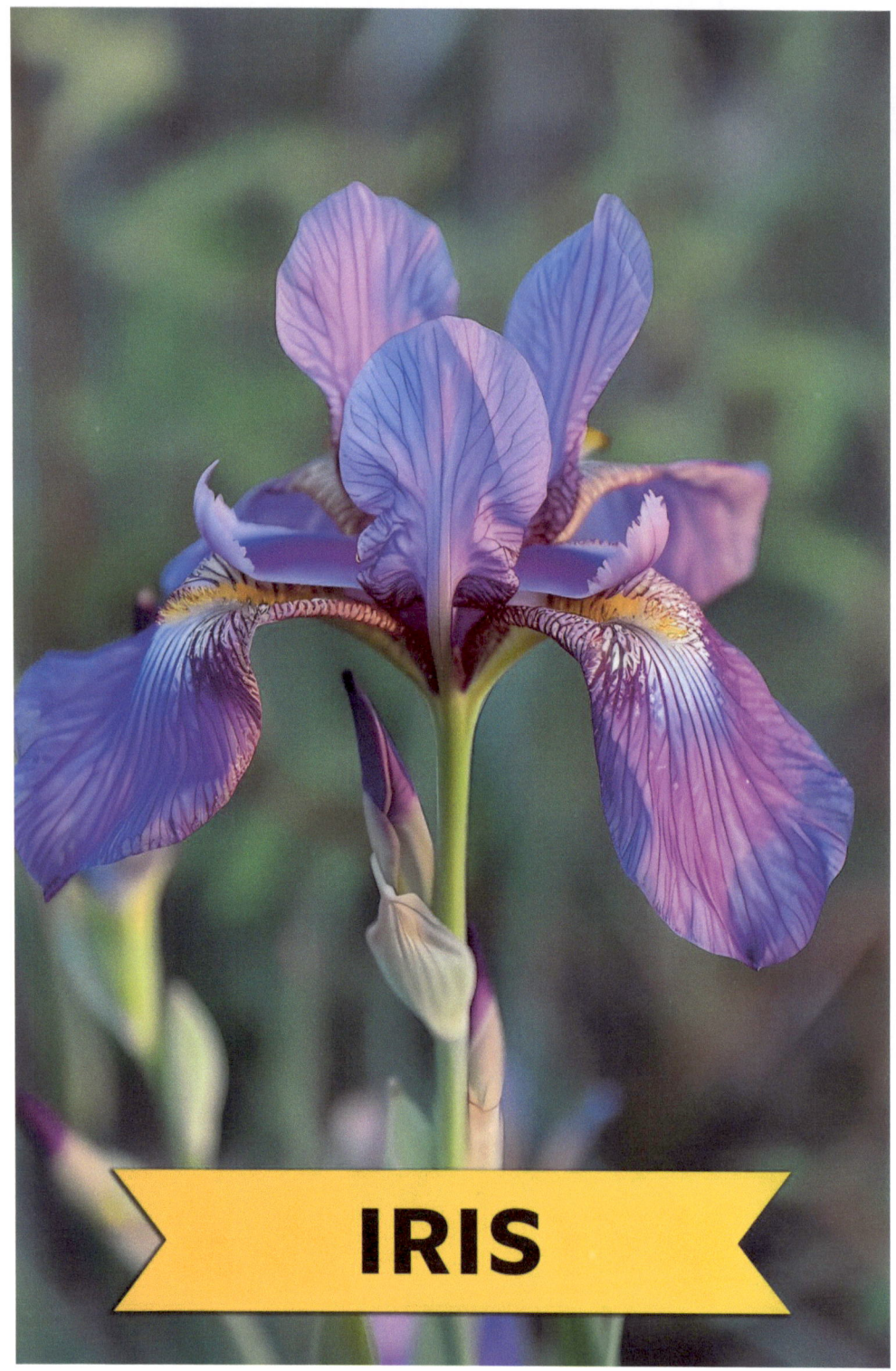

IRIS

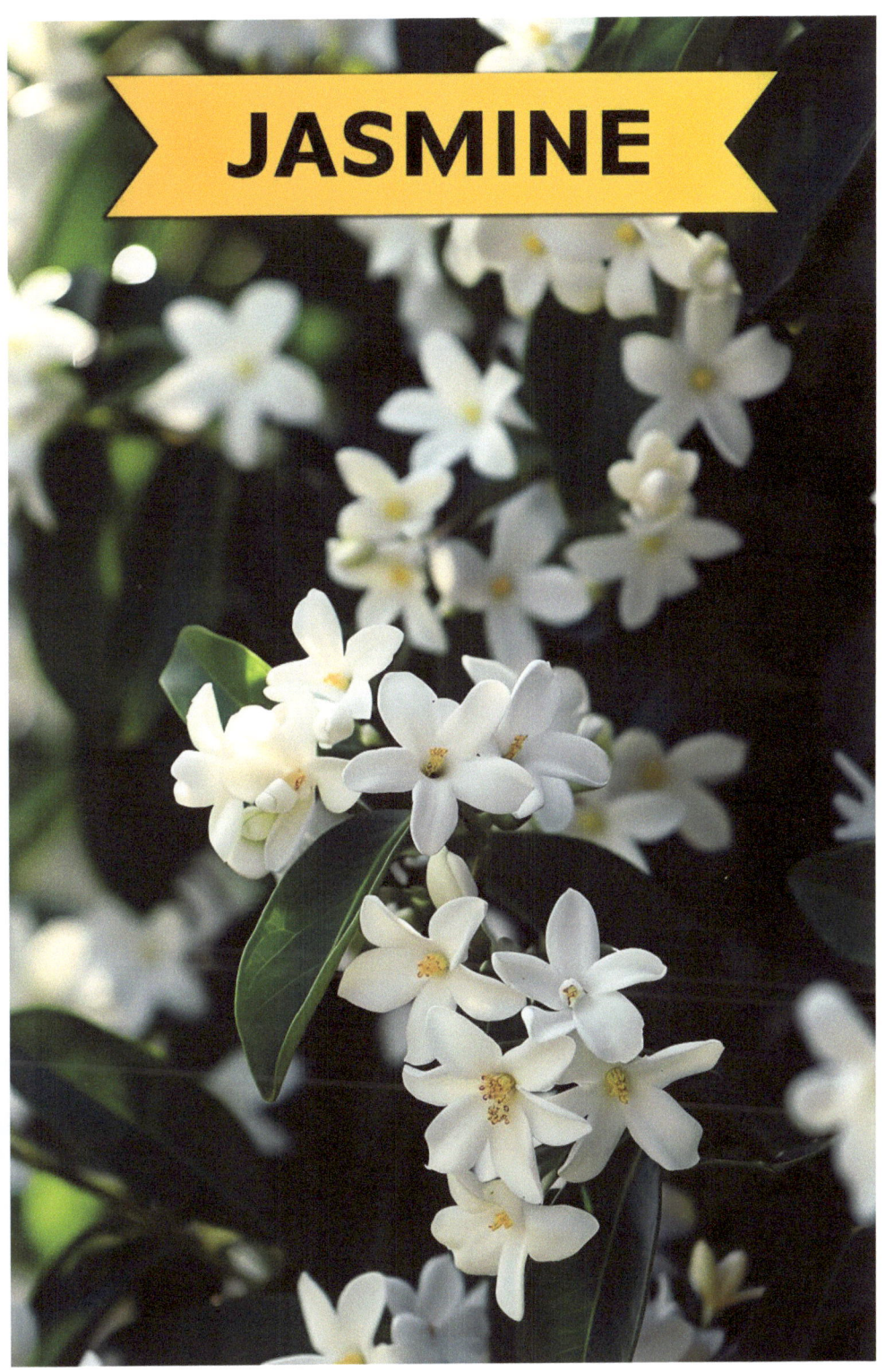

JASMINE

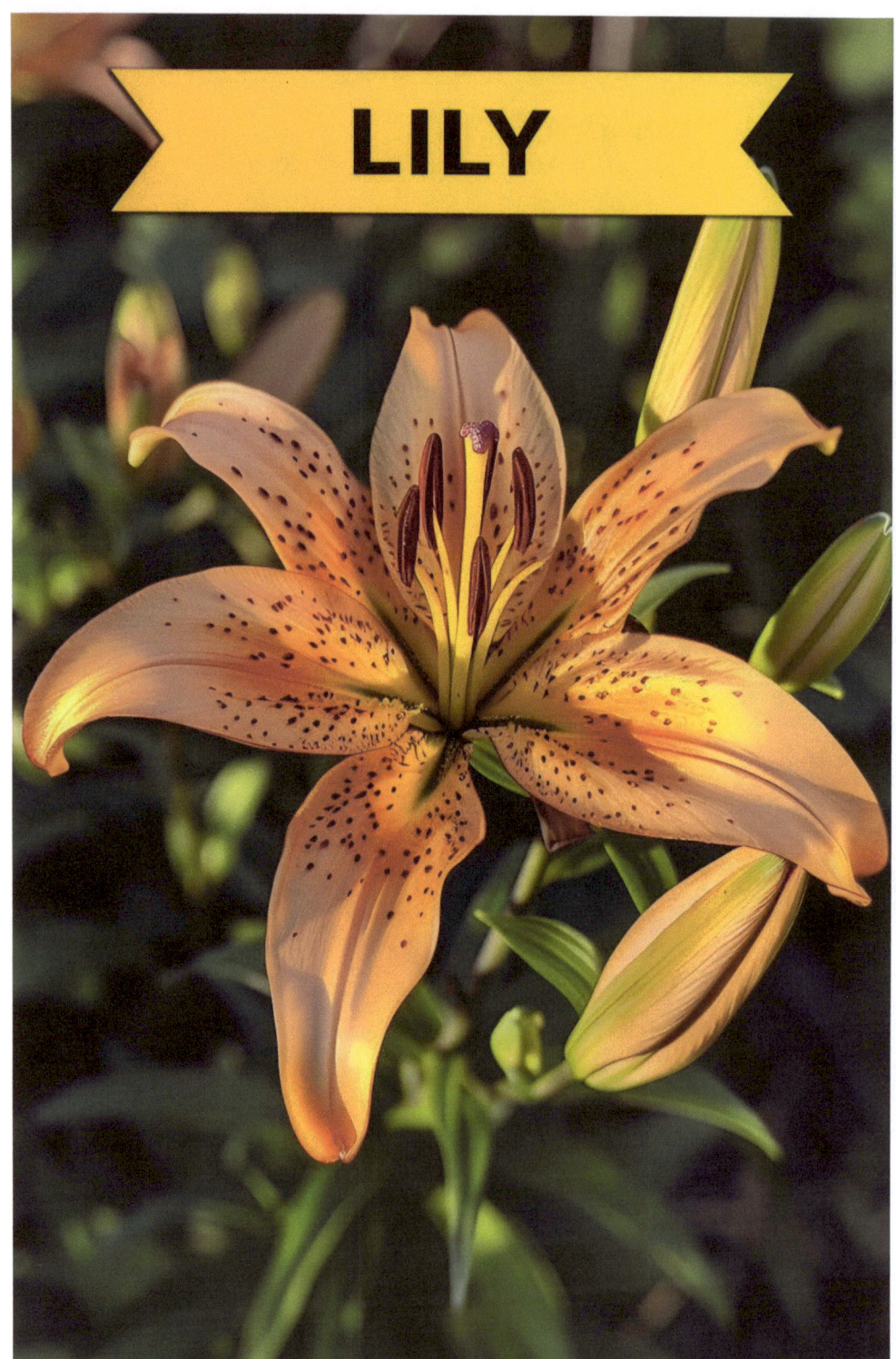

LILY

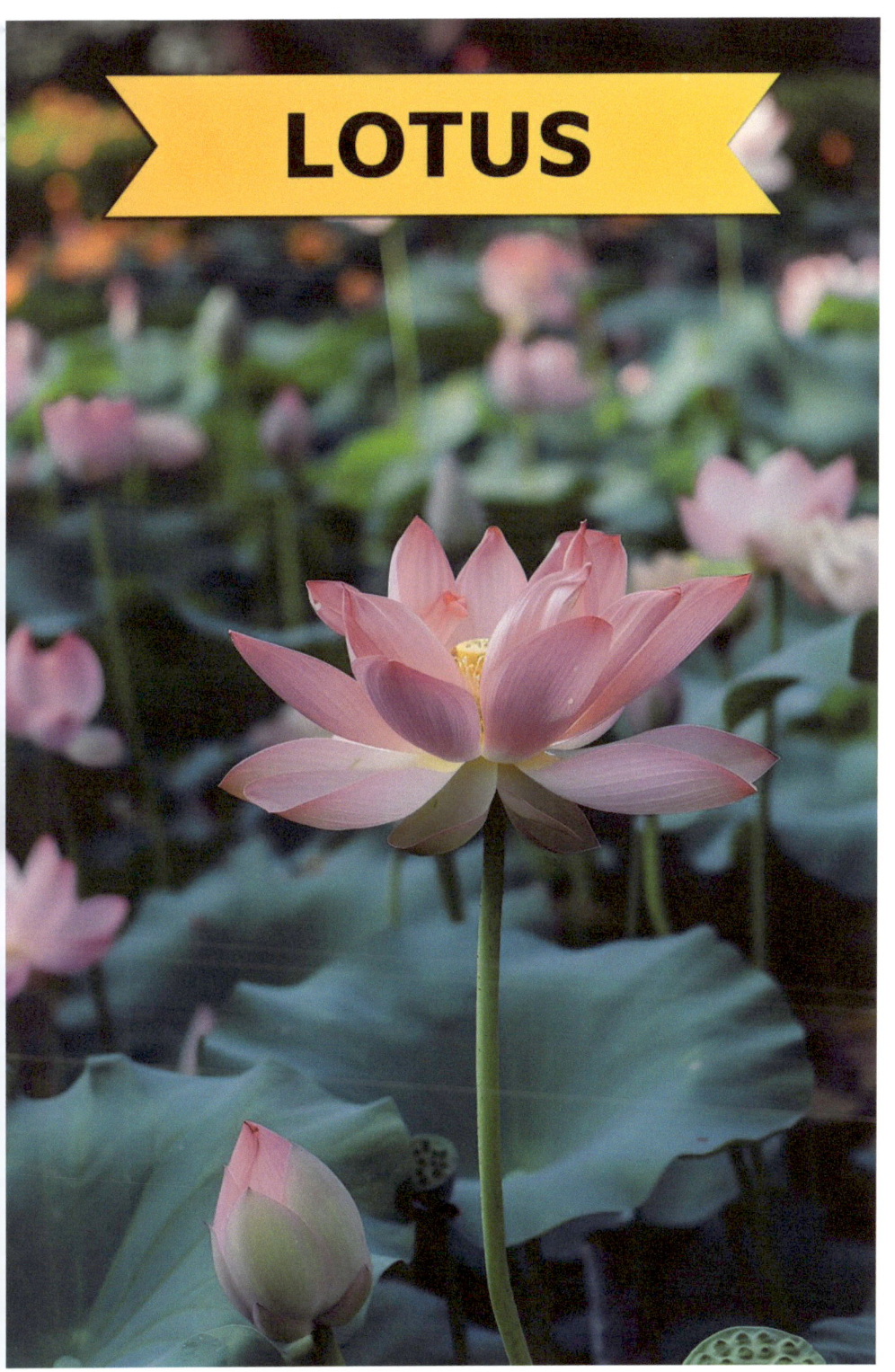

LOTUS

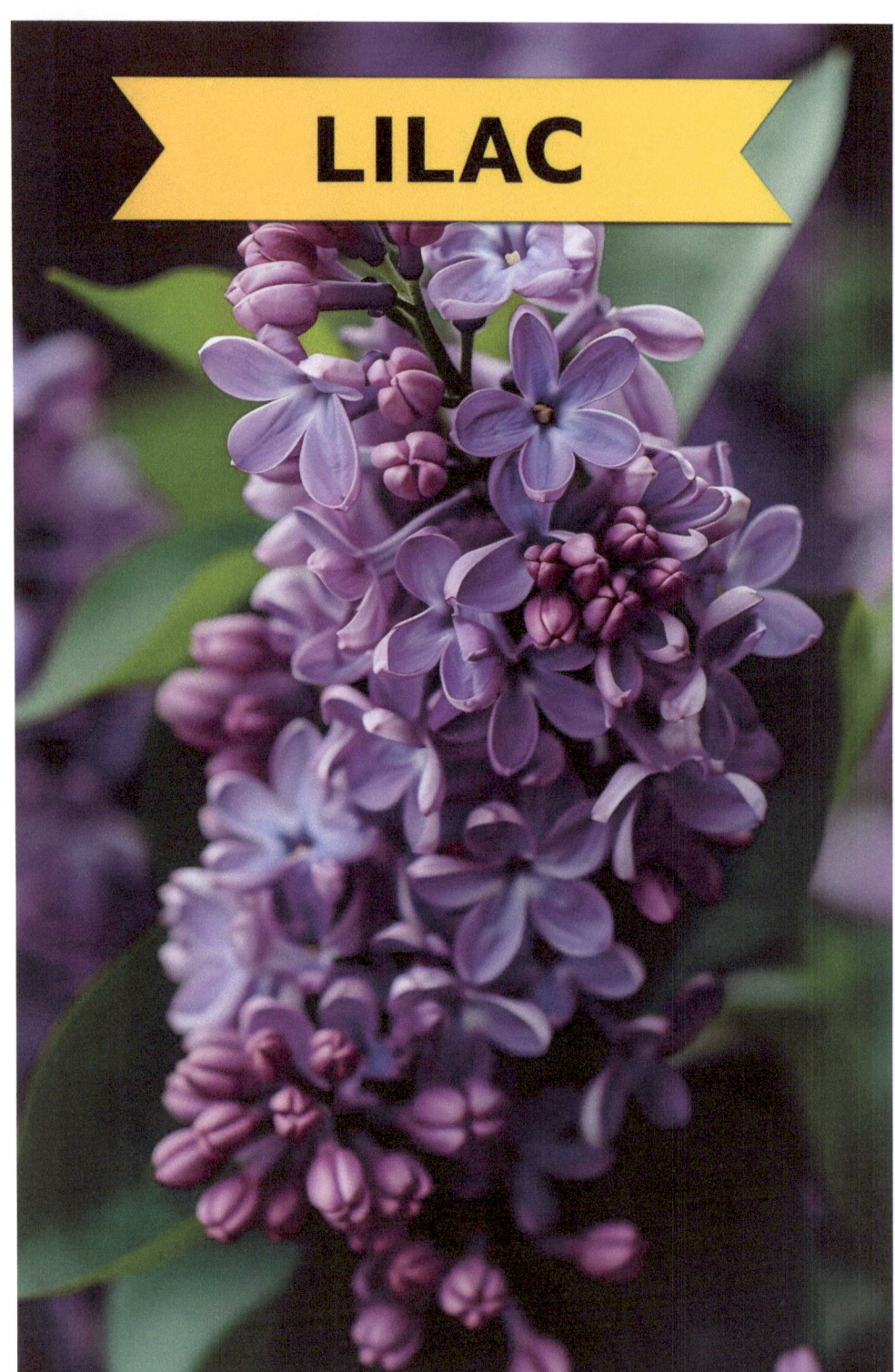

LILAC

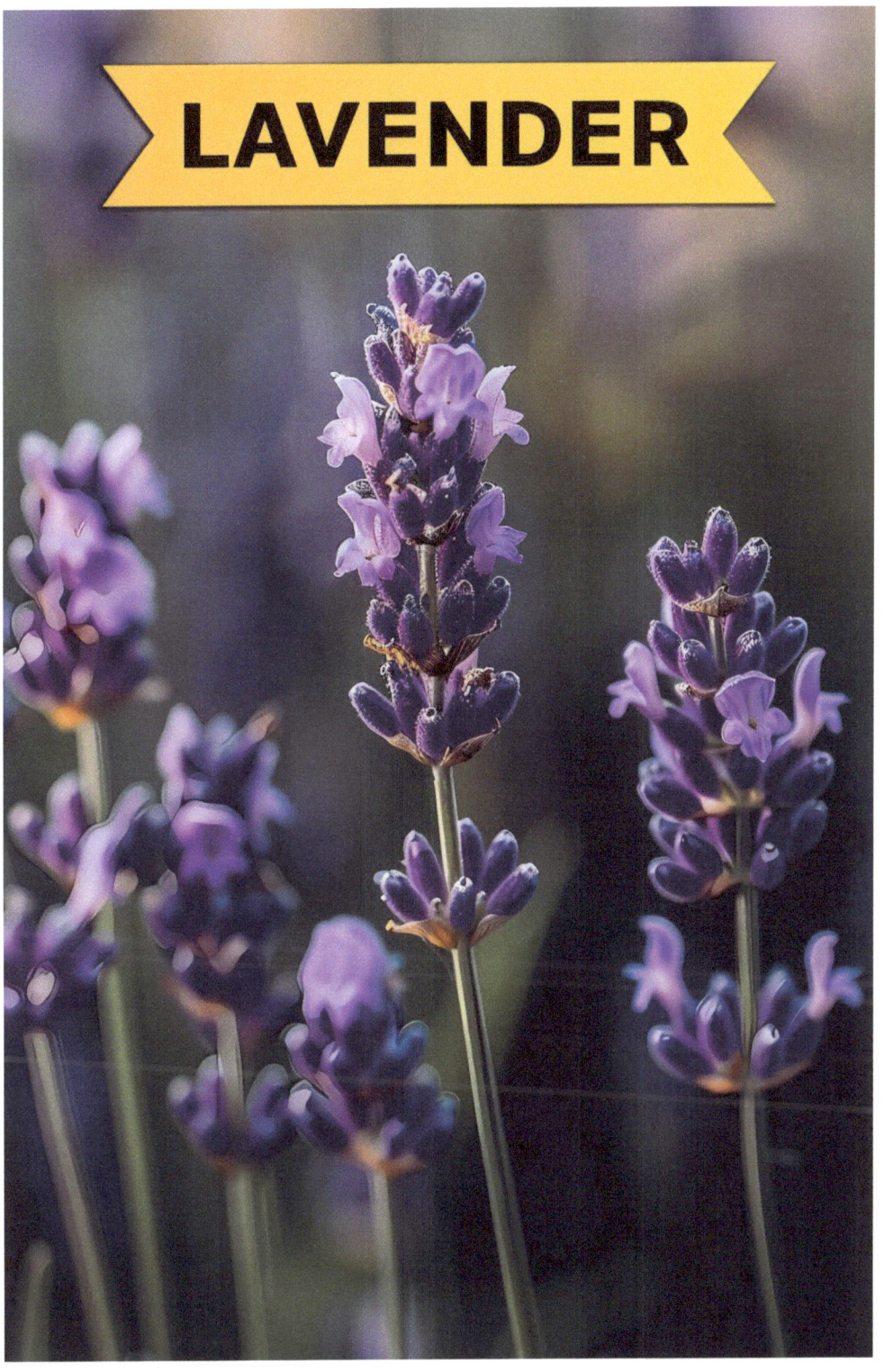

LAVENDER

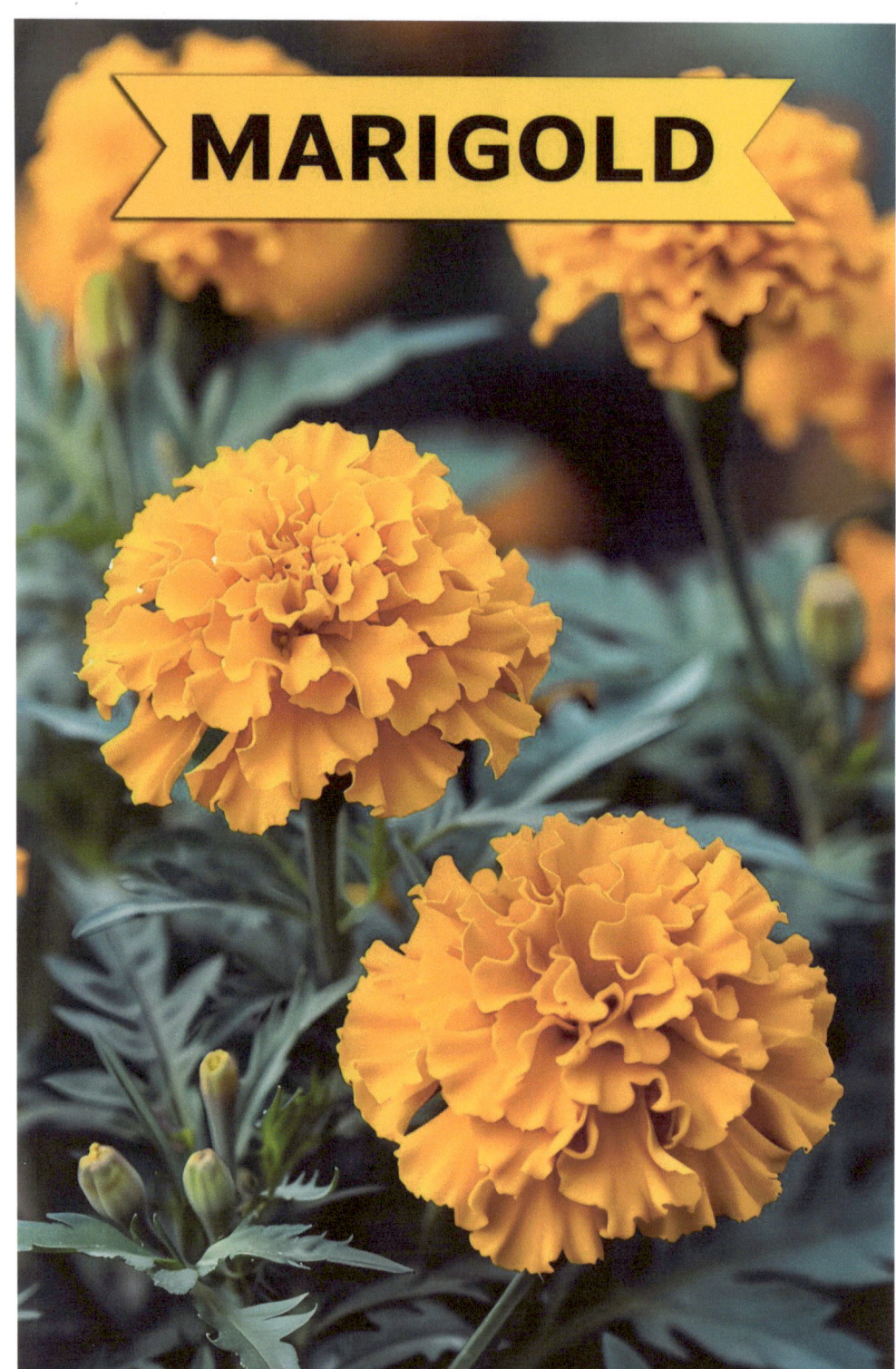

MARIGOLD

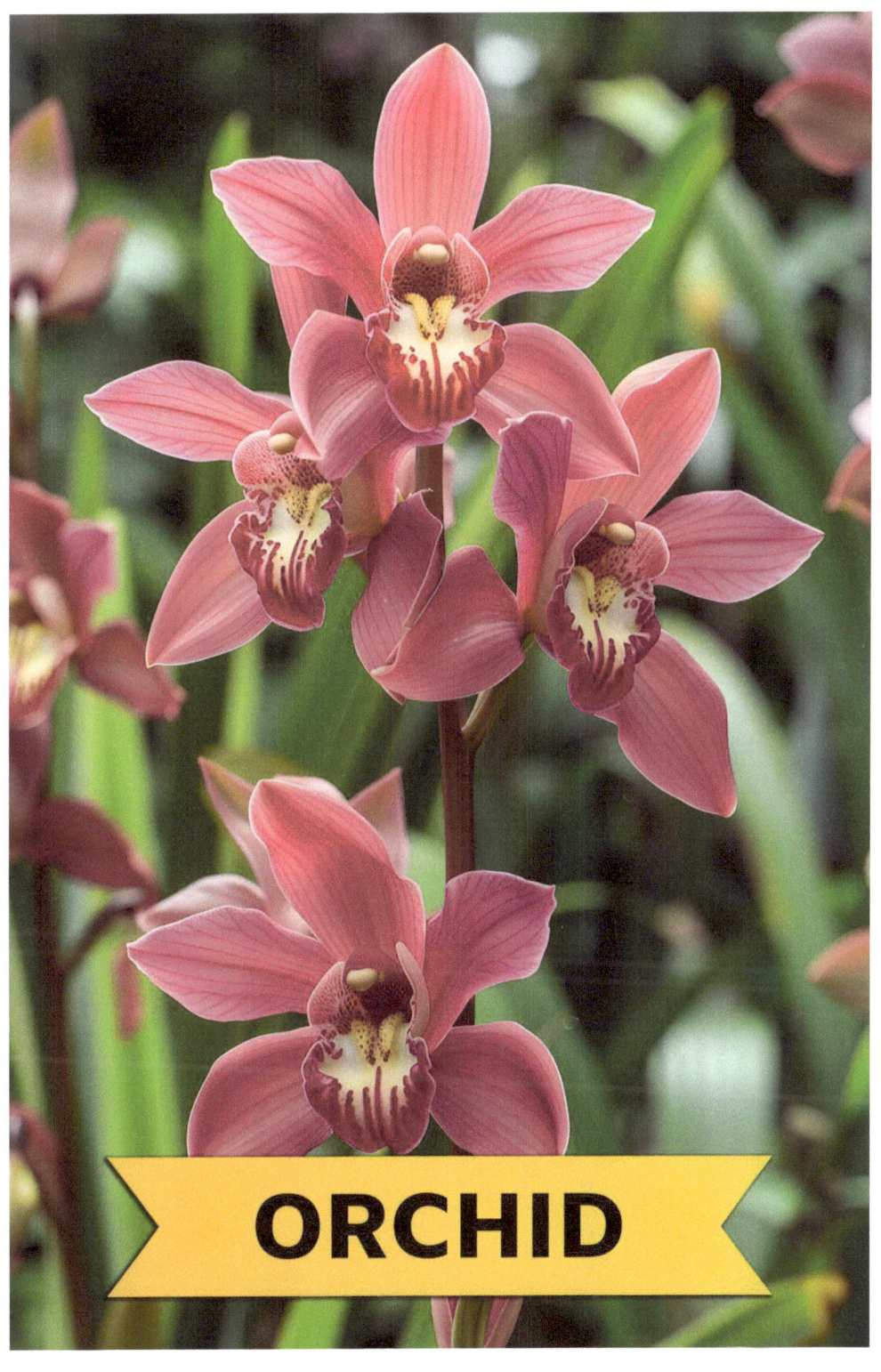

ORCHID

POPPY

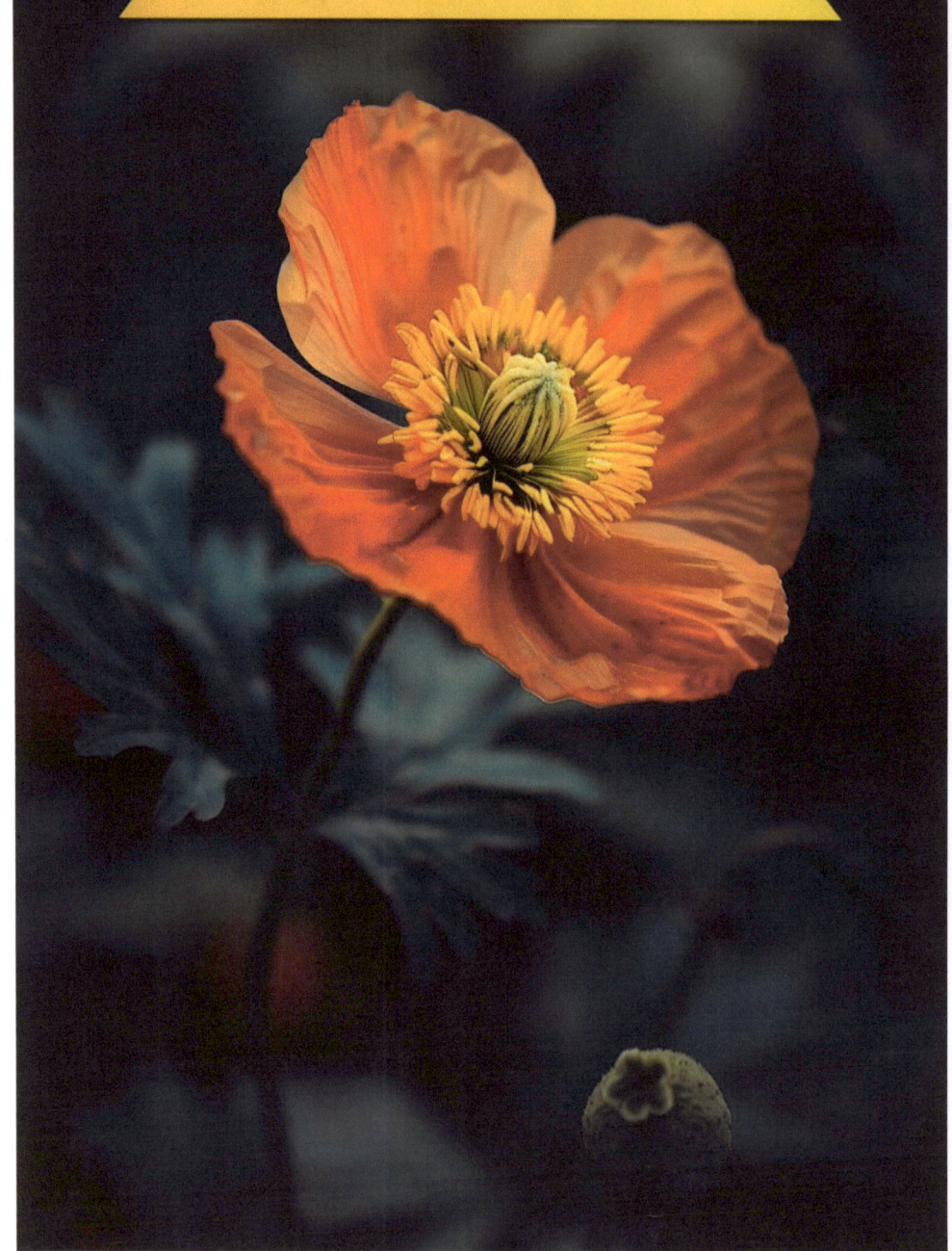

PRIMROSE

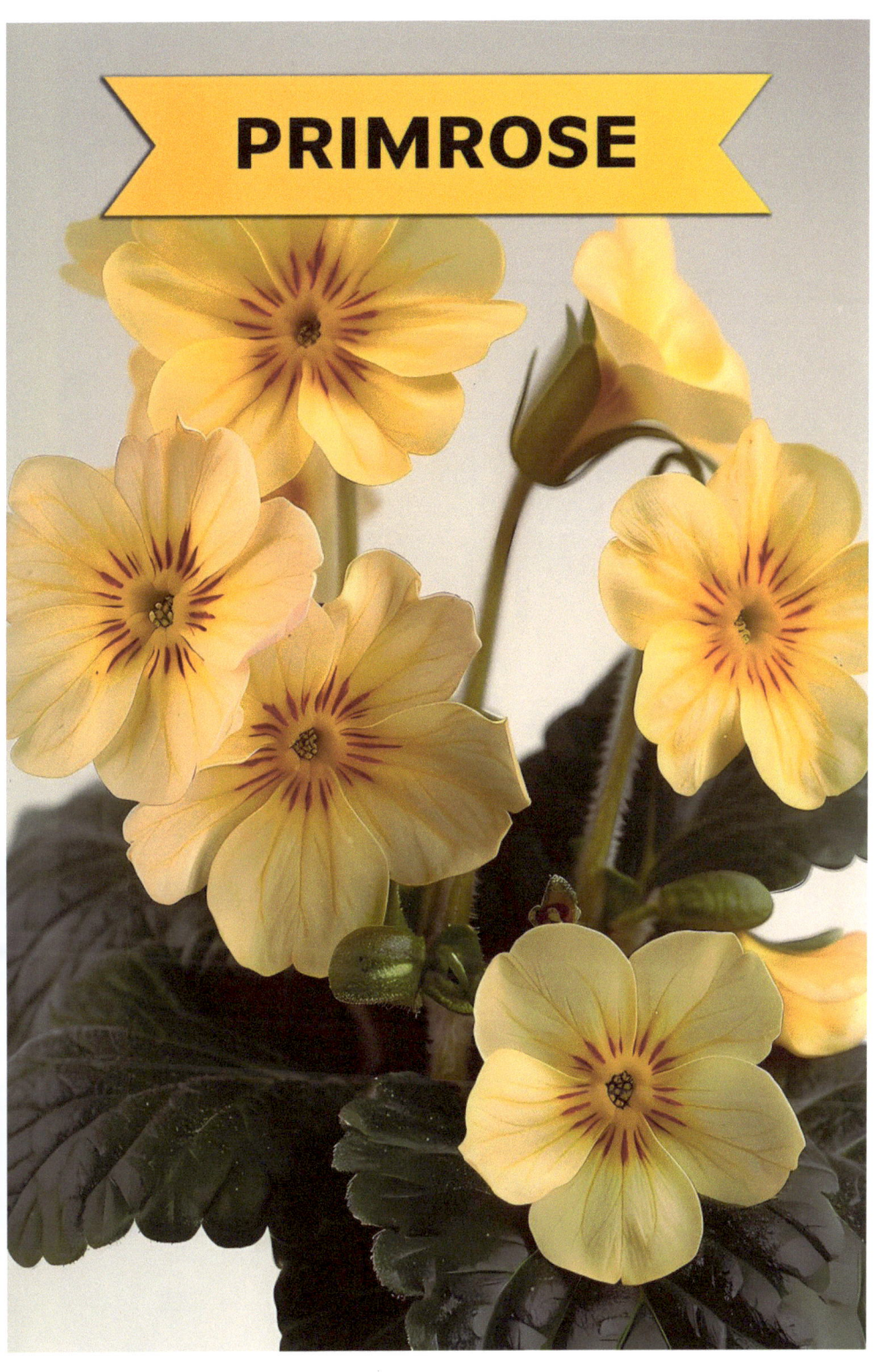

PEONY

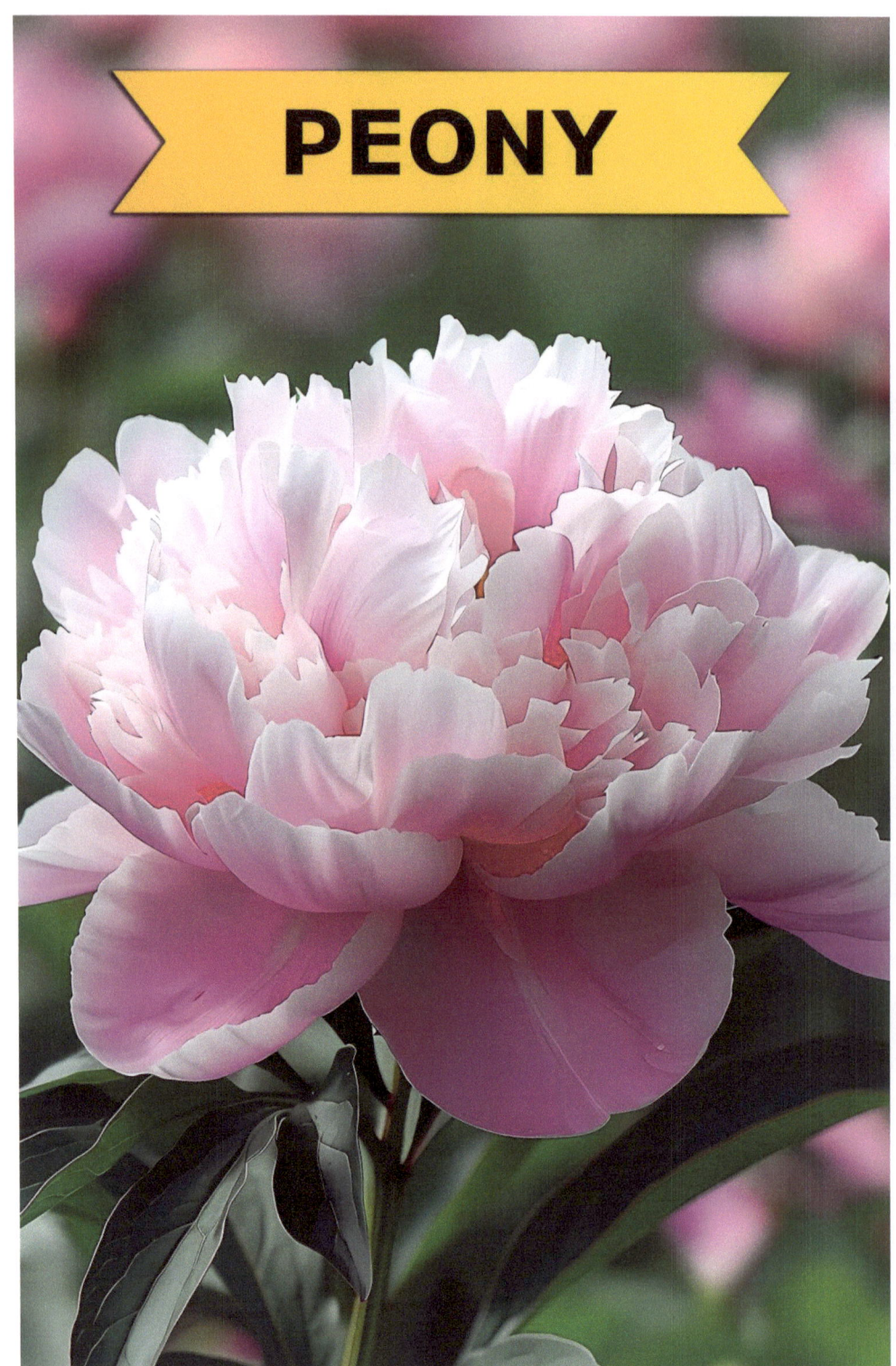

ROSE

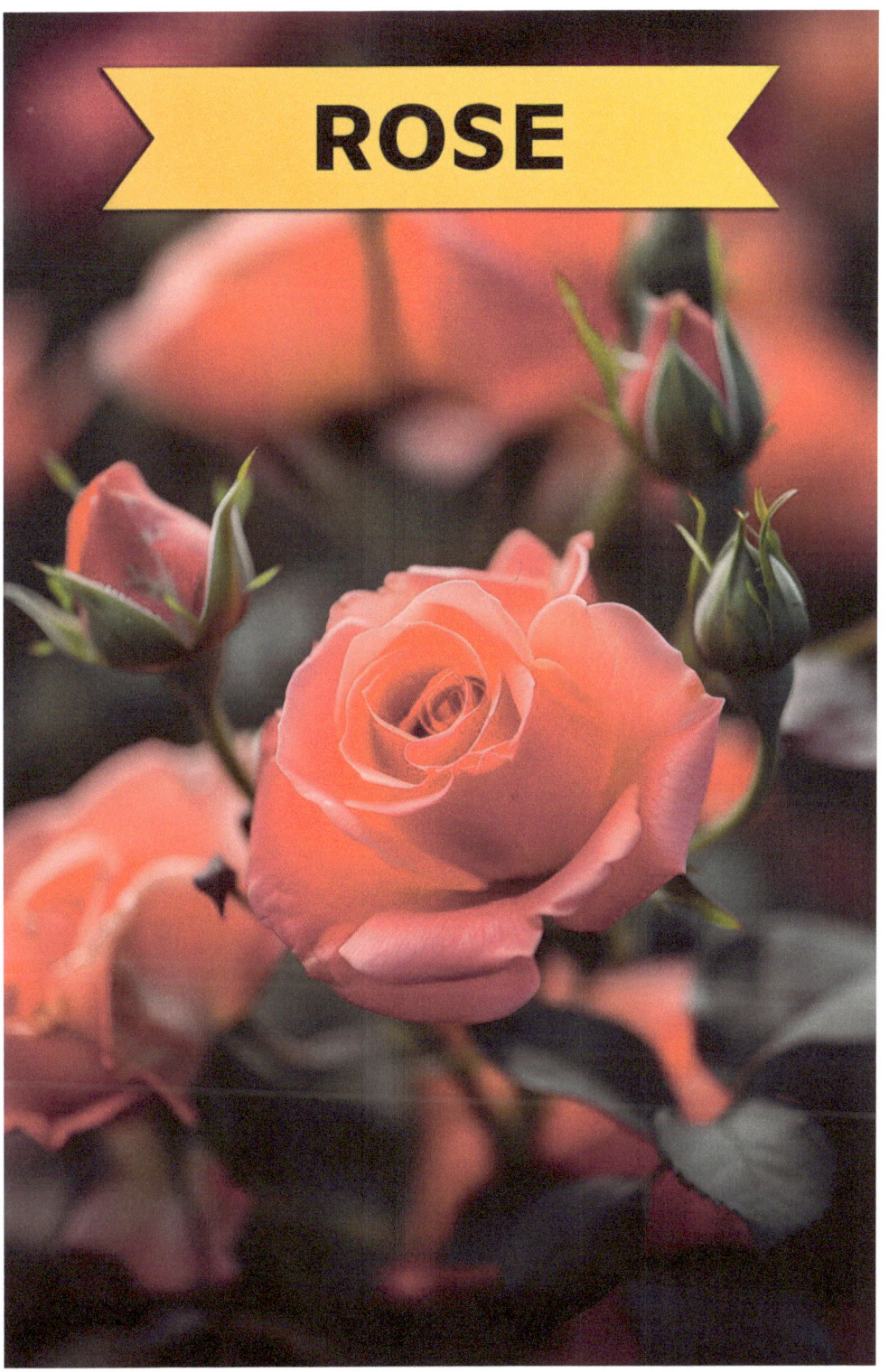

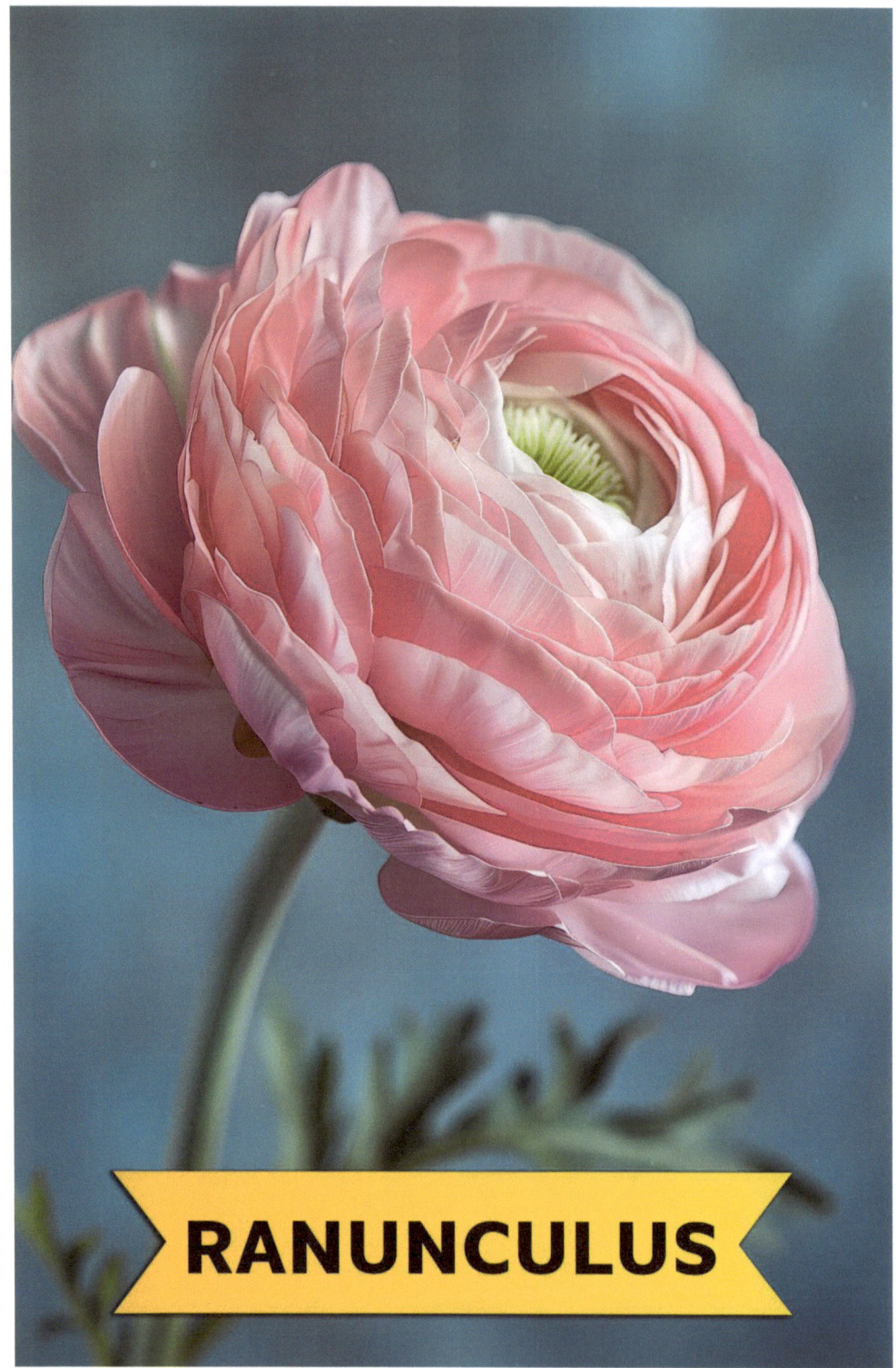

RANUNCULUS

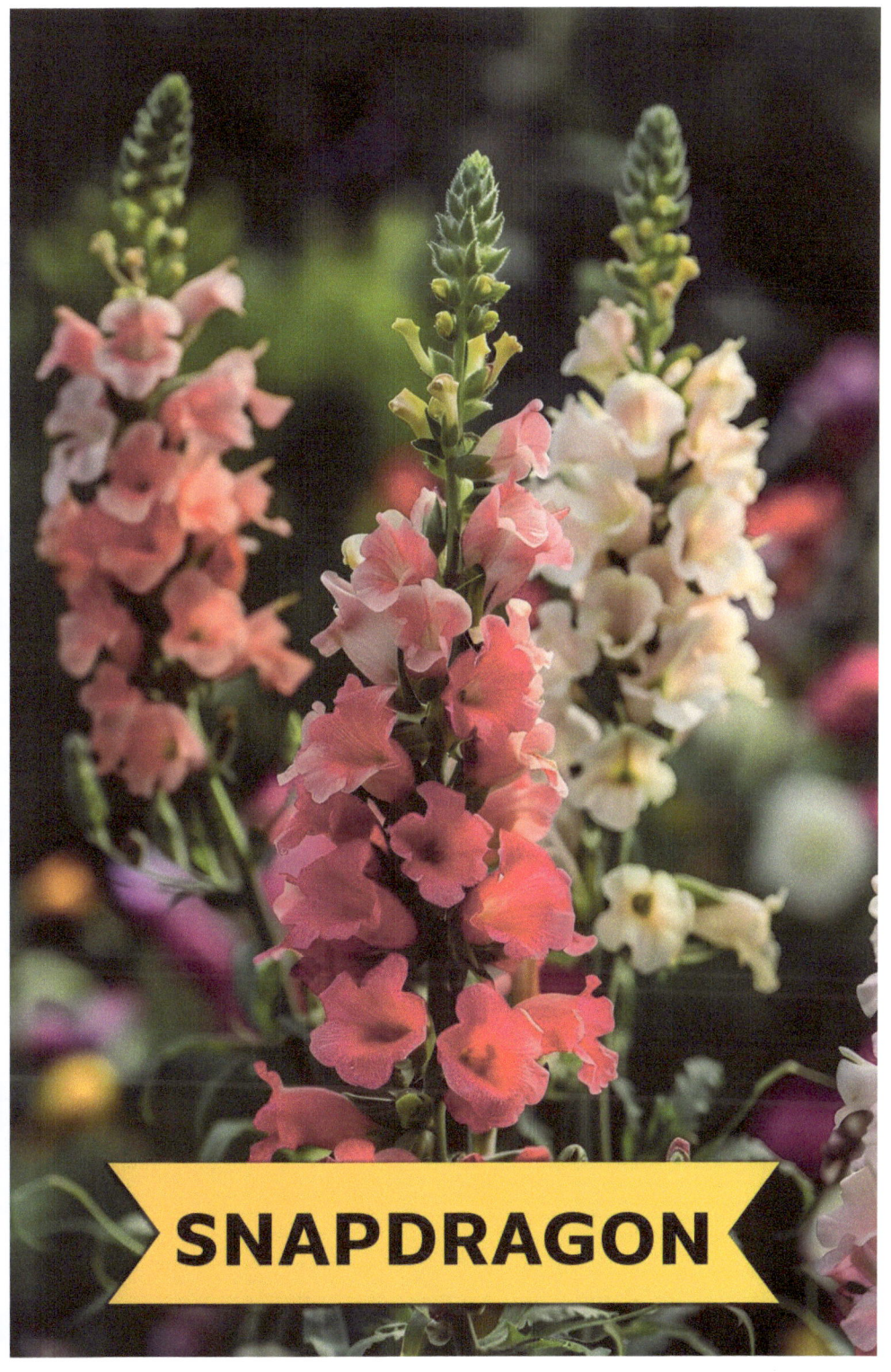

SNAPDRAGON

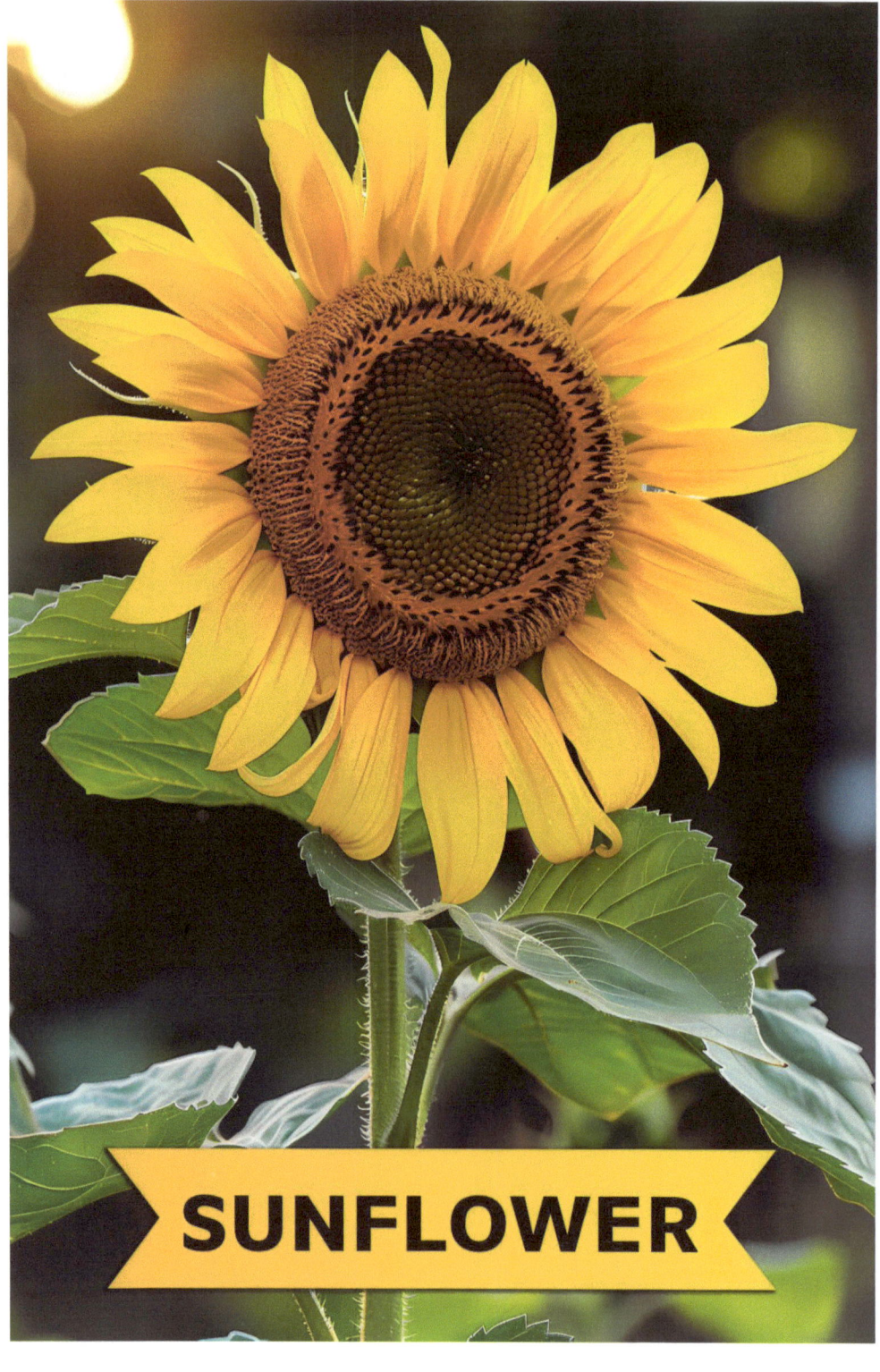

SUNFLOWER

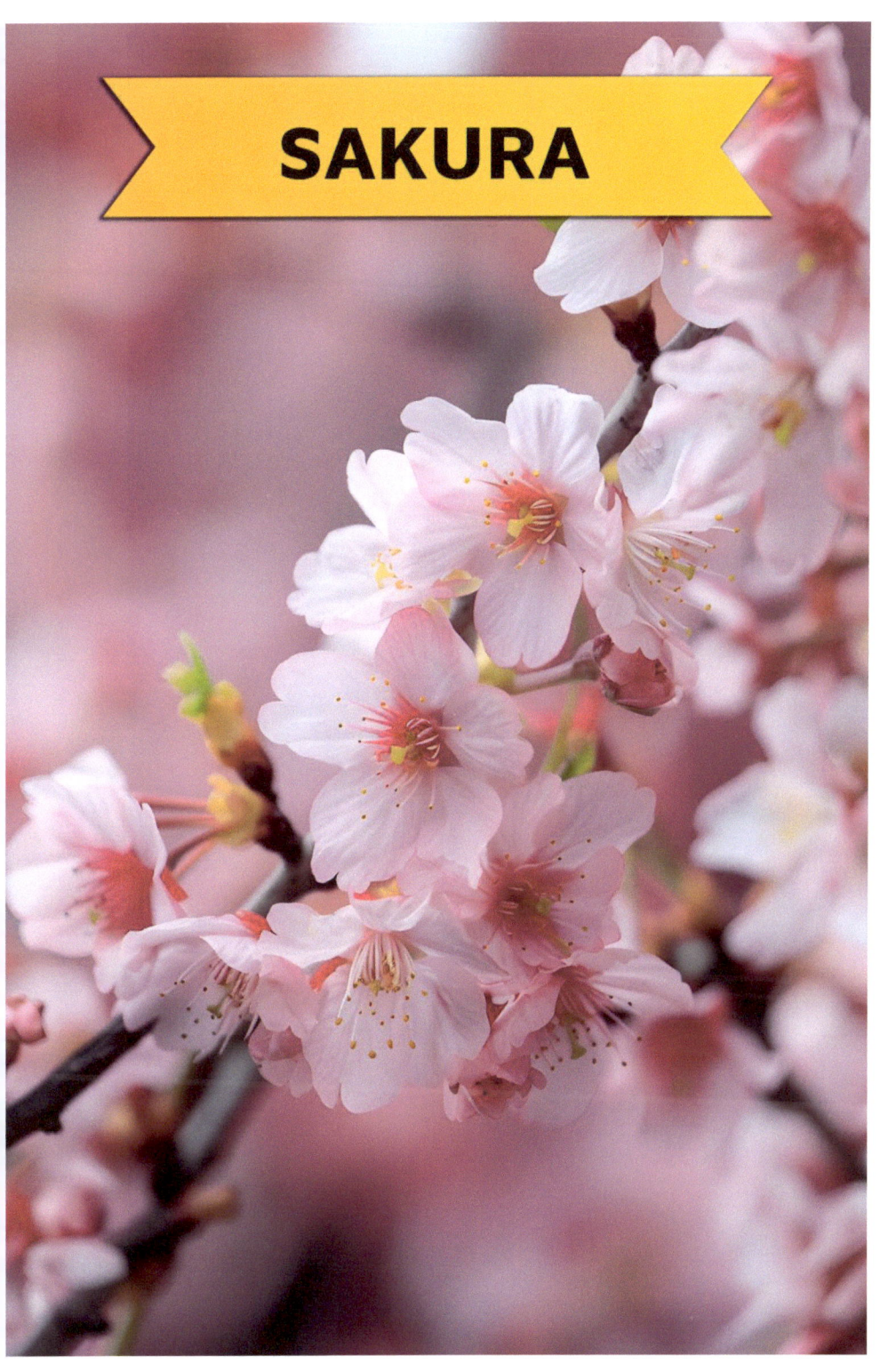

SAKURA

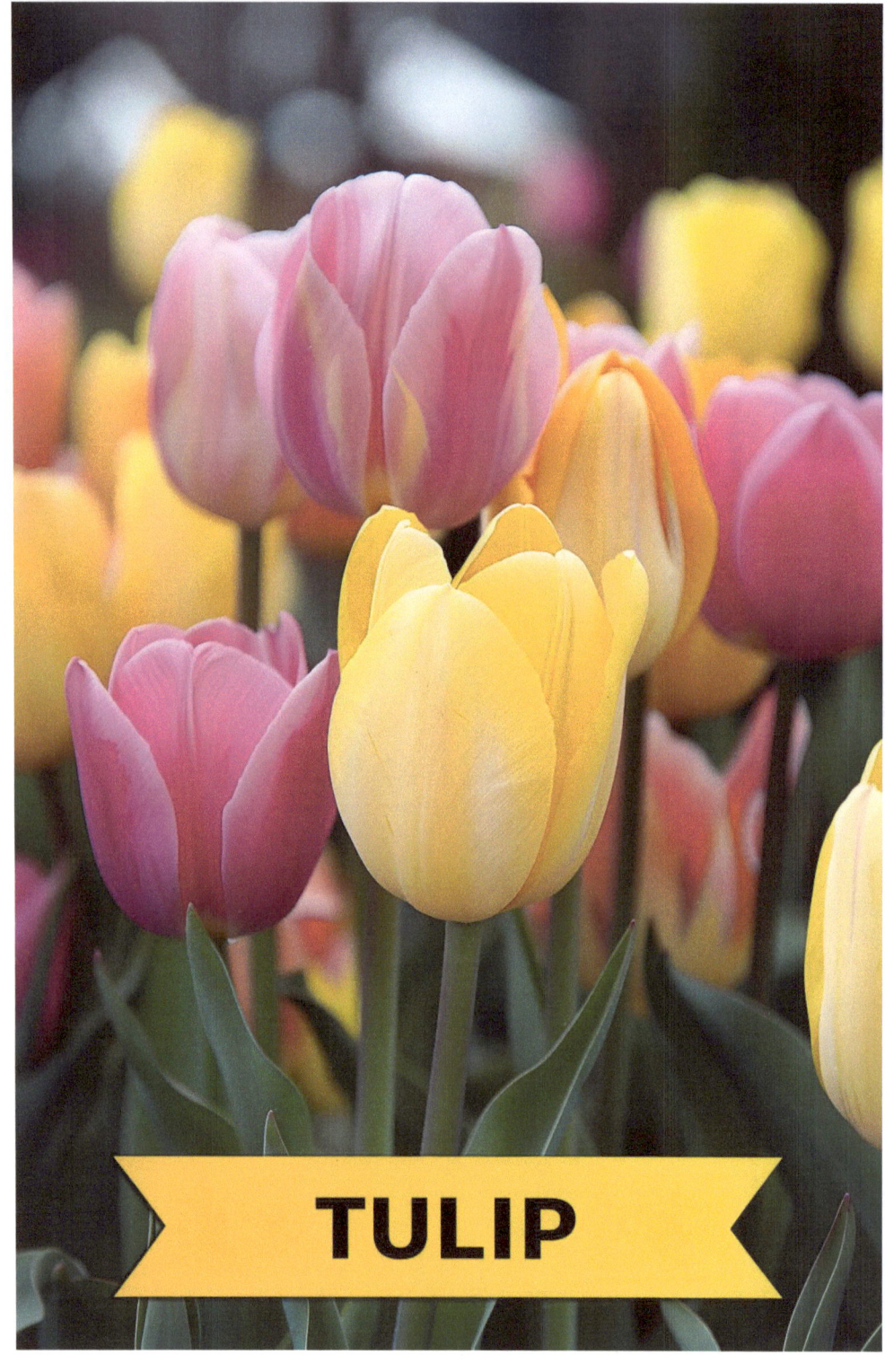

TULIP

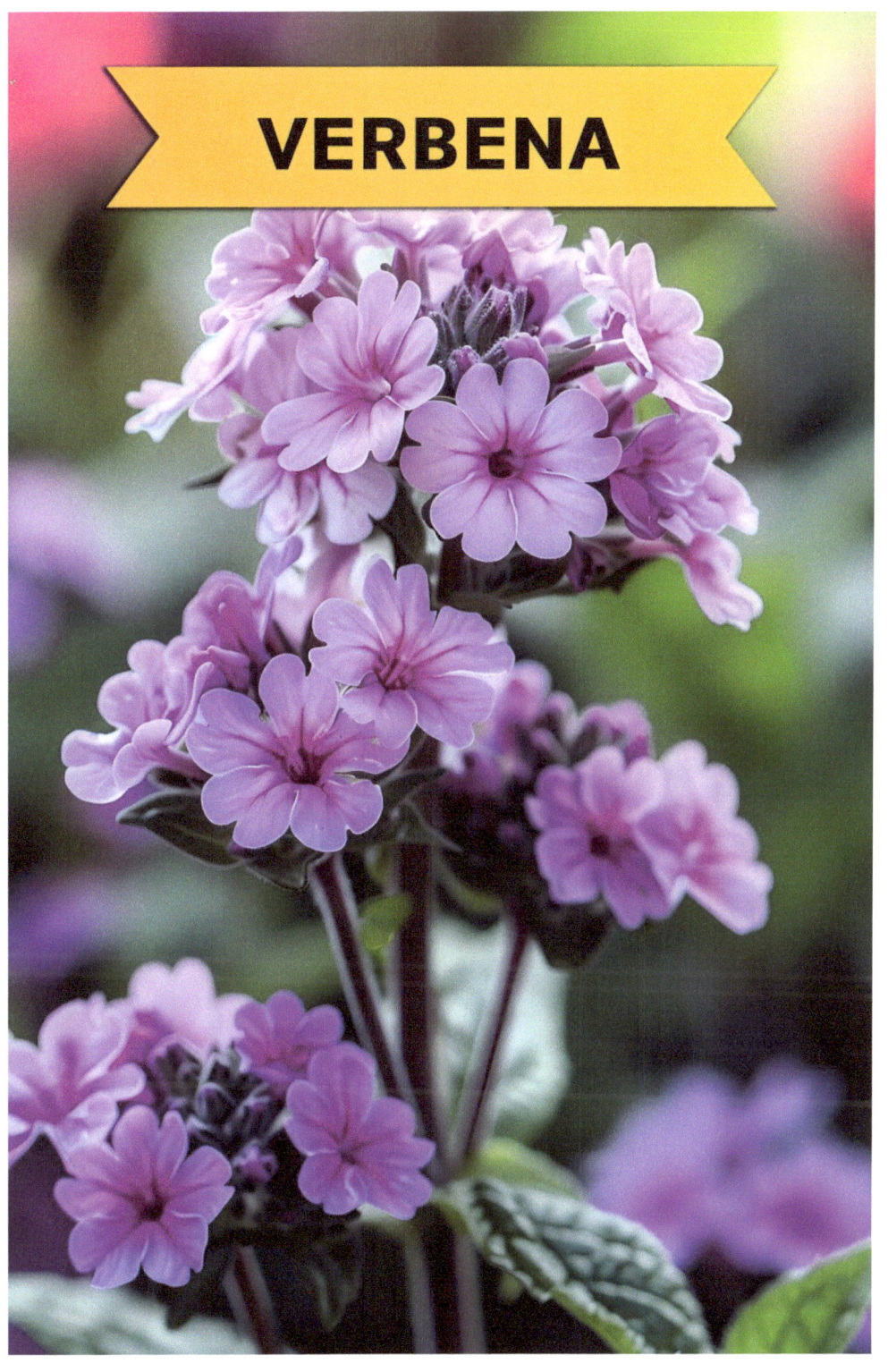

VERBENA

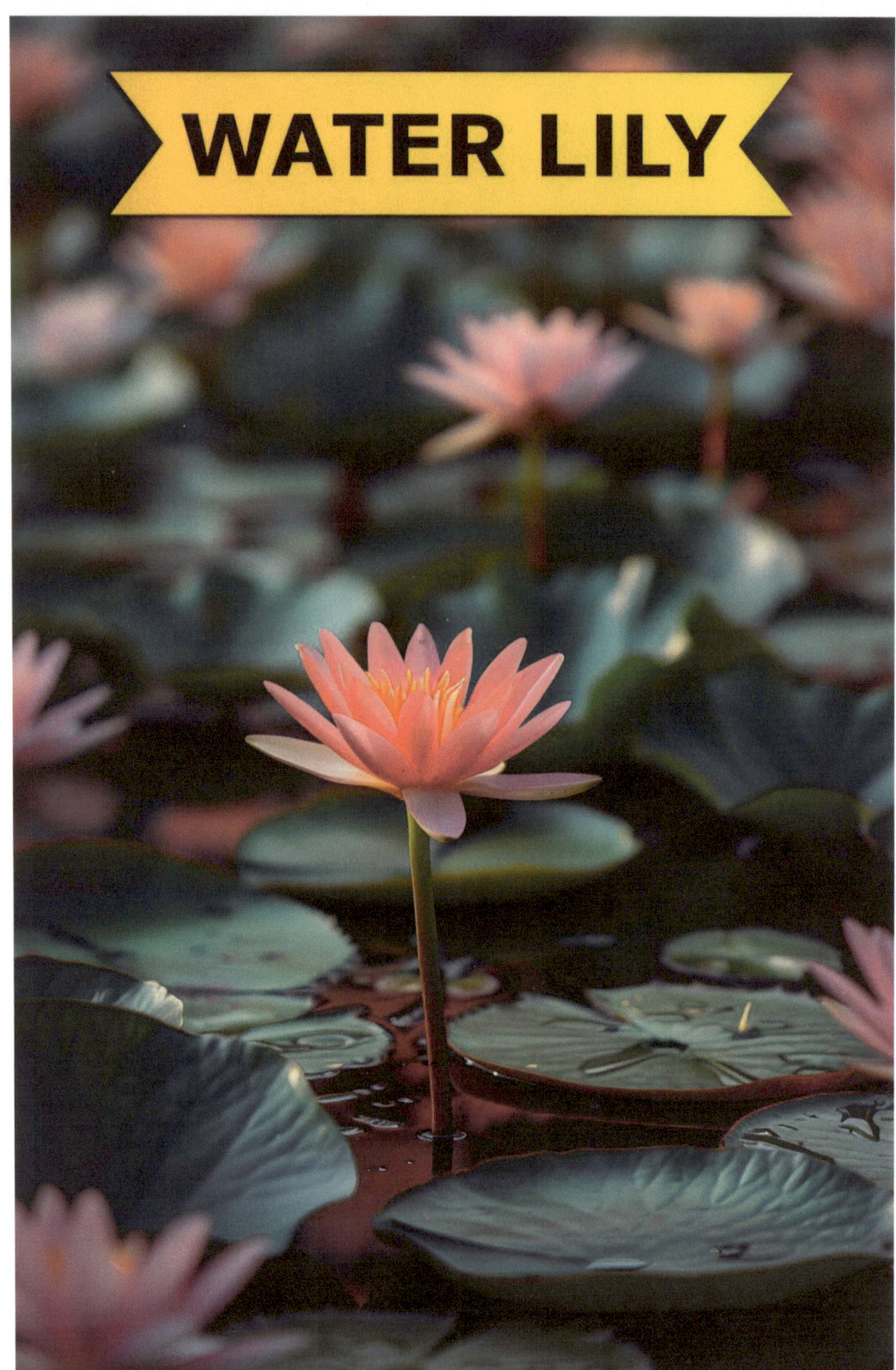

WATER LILY

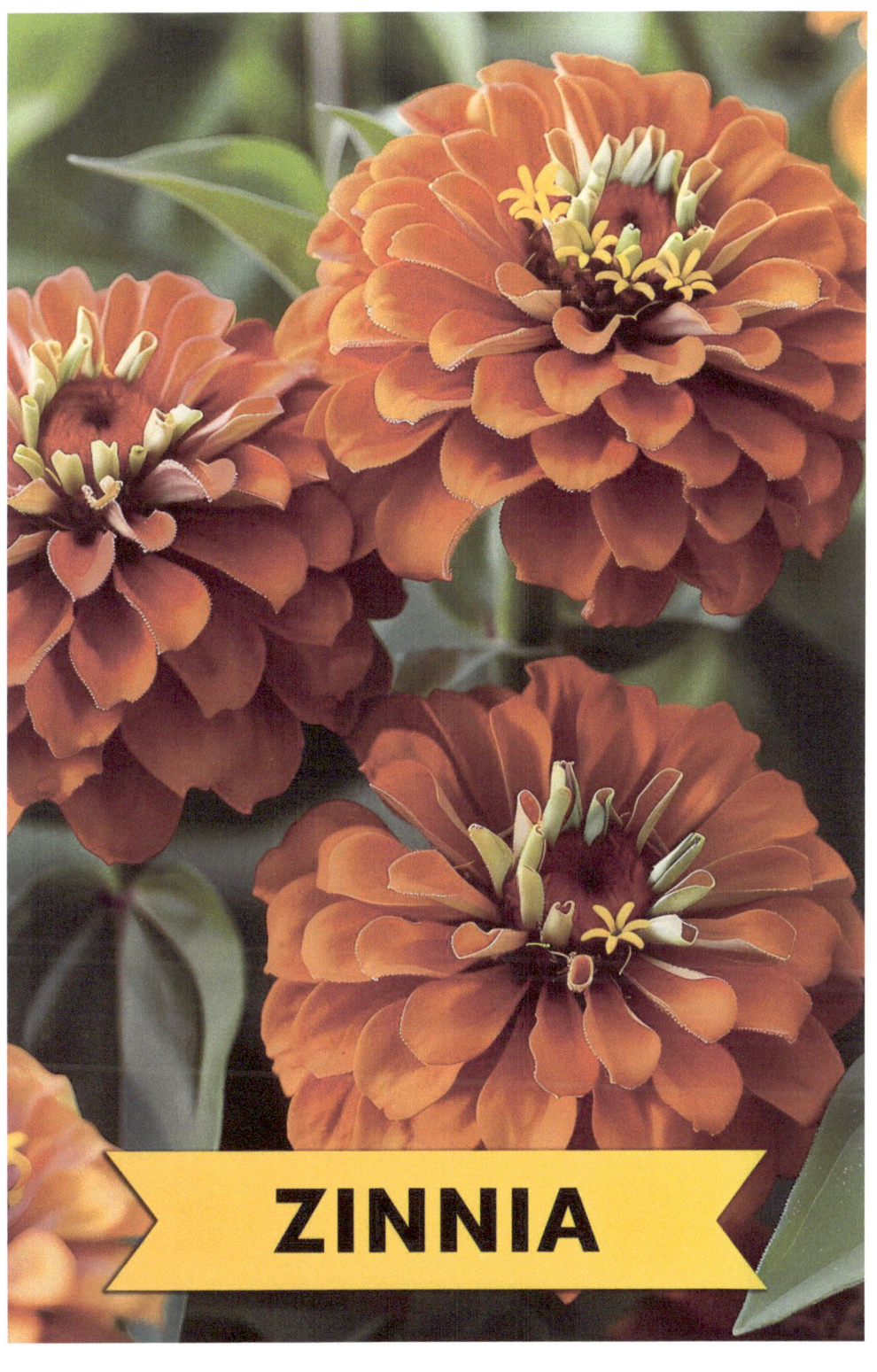

ZINNIA

www.ingramcontent.com/pod-product-compliance
Lightning Source LLC
Chambersburg PA
CBHW040335220526
45473CB00009B/2698